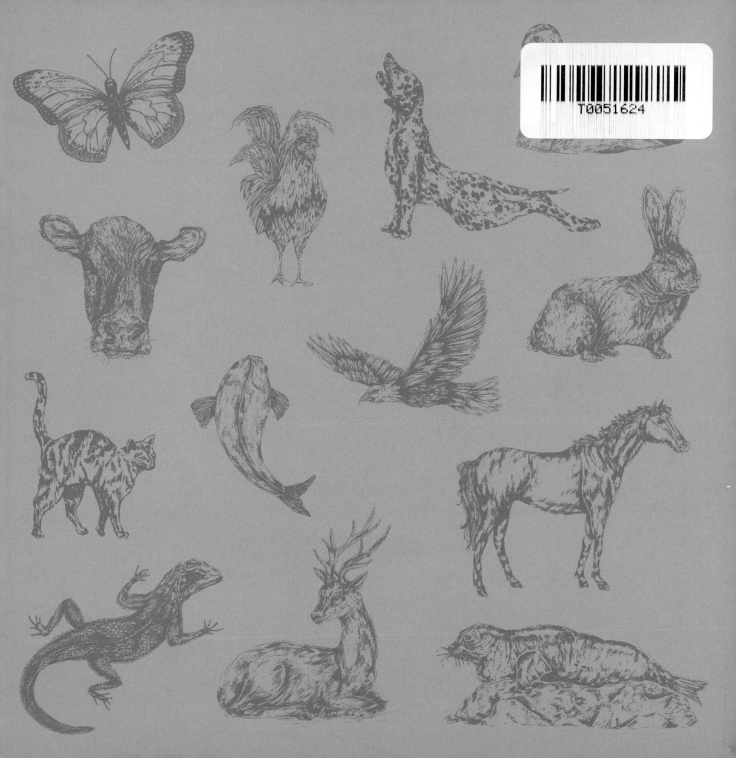

YOGA
ANIMALS

32 Poses from the Wild

First published in Great Britain in 2021 by LOM ART, an imprint of
Michael O'Mara Books Limited
9 Lion Yard
Tremadoc Road
London SW4 7NQ

A CIP catalogue record for this book is available from the British Library.

Papers used by Michael O'Mara Books Limited are natural, recyclable products
made from wood grown in sustainable forests. The manufacturing processes conform
to the environmental regulations of the country of origin.

ISBN: 978-1-912785-49-0 in hardback print format
ISBN: 978-1-912785-50-6 in ebook format

1 2 3 4 5 6 7 8 9 10

This book contains instructions for yoga poses. Every body is different, and
appropriate caution should be used when following these instructions: you
should never attempt to push your body past its limits into painful positions.
Neither the publisher nor the author can accept any liability for any injury or
loss that may occur as a result of information given in this book.

Written by Emily Sharratt
Main animal illustrations and decorations by Jade Mosinski
Design and step-by-step illustrations by Jade Wheaton
Cover design by Natasha Le Coultre
Printed and bound in China
www.mombooks.com

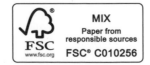

YOGA ANIMALS

32 Poses from the Wild

By Emily Sharratt

Illustrated by Jade Mosinski

LOM ART

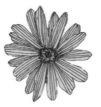

Contents

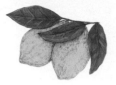

Introduction

Yoga is one of the most popular forms of exercise around the world. There are many different styles or schools, thousands upon thousands of ashrams, shalas and studios, and hundreds of millions of practitioners; increasing numbers of teacher training courses are on offer and a whole industry is built around it. For some, it is simply that: a form of exercise. Others ascribe and adhere to yoga philosophy in a more holistic or integrated way – studying the texts and scriptures, practising not only physical (*hatha*) yoga but also breath work, meditation and mindfulness, and trying to live by the ethics, beliefs and tenets outlined in texts such as Patanjali's *Yoga Sutras*.

This book looks at the physical poses (*asanas*) as well as some breath work (*pranayama*), focusing on those practices that take their name and inspiration from the animal kingdom. From the sweet and soothing hum of bee breath, and the fluid but powerful play of dolphin pose, to the aerial adventures of arm balances such as crow, rooster and feathered peacock, the natural world underpins and informs all aspects of a physical yoga practice. Indeed, this close association with nature might hold some of the answers as to why yoga is so popular compared to other physical stretching and strengthening practices.

In our busy modern lives it is all too easy to feel disconnected from nature. By taking the time to practise yoga, to drop into our own nature via the breath, and by observing and celebrating the human body and its incredible capabilities, all the while visualizing and channelling some of the animal kingdom's most extraordinary creatures, we can reassert or simply remind ourselves of that vital connection. We are a part of nature, even if we don't always feel like it. Yoga gives us the opportunity to experience that on tangible and emotional levels.

How to use this book

The format of the book follows the template of a full, well-rounded yoga session, incorporating stretching, strengthening, energizing and calming elements, while drawing on a number of different yoga styles, from *vinyasa* flows to more static yin poses.

So, if settling in for some solo practice at home, you could use the book as a guide, starting with a breath work exercise and gently warming up. You can then move on to a few rounds of sun salutations and a standing sequence, followed by a standing balance pose; then choose one option from the seated twists, hip-openers, forward folds, back bends, inversions and arm balances, before winding down to a final relaxation. If you have plenty of time, and are feeling especially energetic and ambitious, you could attempt all the poses in the book! On the other hand, you could of course choose one or two poses to focus on, but do make sure you warm up thoroughly. It is also best not to begin any strenuous or advanced yoga practice without in-person guidance from an instructor. Please be especially mindful if working with any injuries or illnesses – in these instances, medical advice should be sought first. I occasionally suggest alternative poses to the ones described. There isn't space in this book to cover them, but you can easily find them online. It is sometimes argued that the purpose of a physical or *asana*-based yoga practice is to prepare the body and mind for meditation. If you have a meditation practice or would like to cultivate one, you may wish to include a seated meditation at the end of your book-led session.

Breath Work

pranayama

An important part of the physical practice of yoga is breath work or *pranayama*. The Sanskrit *pranayama* comes from the word 'prana', meaning 'life force' or 'energy', and refers to the use of the breath to control or channel that energy. Indeed, some argue that the word 'yoga' itself – which comes from the Sanskrit meaning 'to yoke' – refers to the connection of body and mind via the breath.

The benefits of regular yoga breath work can be physical, mental, emotional and energetic – from strengthening and toning all the muscles of the respiratory system and increasing lung capacity, to enhancing the quality of sleep through the ability to relax properly. It flushes away stale air from the body, improving circulation and therefore the efficiency of the digestive and eliminatory systems, and assists with the removal of toxins. When anxiety manifests itself in your body, it can often cause shallow, upper-chest breathing.

But slow deep breathing that goes all the way into the abdomen – by fully expanding the lungs and therefore flattening the respiratory diaphragm – can help to slow the heart rate, and send the message to the sympathetic nervous system (sometimes known as the 'fight or flight' reflex) that it is not needed at this moment. This in turn allows the parasympathetic nervous system (often referred to as the 'rest and the digest' response) to activate. *Pranayama* is a pathway to a deeper yoga practice, allowing the yogi to access more challenging poses (*asanas*) and a stiller mind.

Breath work can be practised at different points of a yoga session depending on what *pranayama* exercise one is doing and what the desired effects are. However, one or more exercise is often performed at the start of a session in order to calm, energize and connect with the body, while quietening the mind.

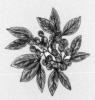

Bee Breath
bhramari

Bhramar is the Sanskrit word for 'bee', and this breathing exercise takes its name from the humming sound made on the exhalation – like a happy bee busy collecting nectar. It is a great way to start your yoga session, using sound to gently draw the mind away from its chatter, bringing awareness to the body and breath.

We are all aware of the vital importance of bees to the continuation of life on earth. Bees also represent community, because each bee works for the good of its whole colony, and when practising bee breath in a group class or session, the sounds of the individual hums often blend together in a way that is reminiscent of this. Even practising this breath exercise alone can bring an awareness of this interconnectivity.

Bee Breath Pose Step by step

This audible breath helps to focus and soothe the mind, as well as lengthening the natural exhalation, which makes space for a fuller, deeper inhalation.

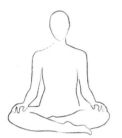

1 Come to a comfortable position, either seated cross-legged, kneeling or with legs extended if that is more accessible for you. You can use a yoga block or cushion under the bottom to lift up out of the hips and allow the pelvis to tilt and the thigh bones to descend. Lift the crown of the head towards the sky while letting the tailbone draw towards the earth.

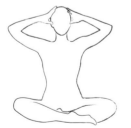

2 If it feels comfortable for you, use your thumbs to gently close your ears, wrapping the other fingers round the back of the head. Let your eyes and lips close, too.

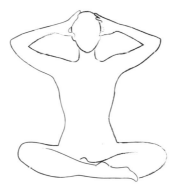

3 Inhale through the nose. As you exhale, keeping the lips closed, release the breath in a long *mmm* sound. This can be at whatever volume and pitch feels natural for you. Keep the sound going to the very end of the exhalation.

4 Repeat at least twice more, but you can carry on for as long as feels nice.

5 When you've finished, continue to sit with your eyes closed, feeling the vibration of the sound in your head. Observe how you feel.

Lion

simhasana

While technically a physical pose (*asana*), the most recognizable
and arguably the most important part of lion posture – which
is described in the circa tenth- or eleventh-century text,
the *Vimanarcanakalpa* – is the roar-like breath.

When combined with the wide-open mouth, the extended
tongue and the rolling eyes, *simhasana* is supposed to resemble
the ferocious king of the beasts, and perhaps bring a sense
of that same power, fearlessness, strength and
energy to the yoga practice.

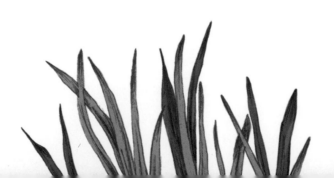

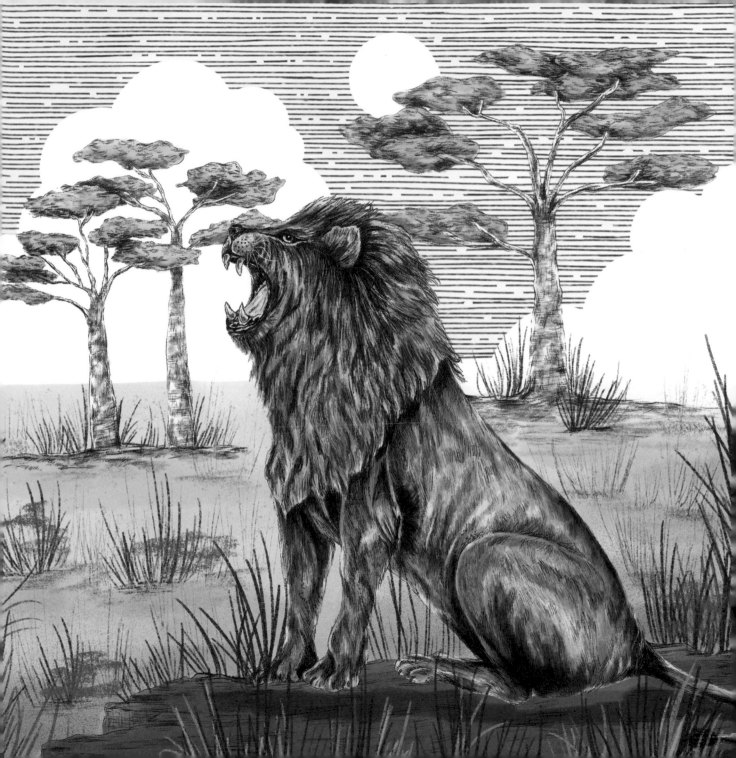

Lion Pose Step by step

A benefit of practising lion pose is its sheer silliness, allowing the yogi to let go of self-consciousness and tensions, and embrace an element of play.

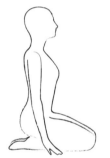

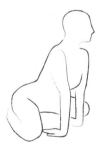

1 Come to a comfortable kneeling position. You can use your mat doubled-up or a blanket beneath the knees to support them, and/or a cushion or block under the bottom to alleviate any pressure. If any kneeling position is uncomfortable for you, choose a different seated position. Place the hands on the floor in front of the knees (knees can be together or slightly apart), fingers spread like claws either pointing towards you (to add a wrist and forearm stretch) or away.

2 Take a deep breath in through the nose.

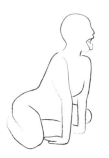

3 Simultaneously open your mouth wide, sticking your tongue out as far as it can go, and open your eyes wide and let the eyeballs roll upwards towards the top of your head, and exhale in a loud, strong, panting *haaaa* sound. Empty the lungs of air, drawing the belly button back to the spine at the end of the exhalation. Feel any tensions, unwanted thoughts or stale energy being expelled with the breath.

4 Repeat at least twice more.

5 When you have finished, kneel or sit with the eyes closed for a couple of natural breaths, observing how you feel and any shifts in energy that might have occurred as a result of this practice.

Cat-cow
marjaryasana-bitilasana

For those new to yoga, these poses might sound like an odd pairing –
cats and cows have very little in common, after all. However, combined,
these two postures are the ideal way to warm and wake up the spine,
moving it through its full range of motion, as well as gently activating
the muscles of the core and hips. Both poses start from a neutral,
kneeling-on-all-fours position. Cow involves dropping the tummy
(almost as though it were a cow's udder!), broadening the collarbone,
opening the chest and looking up. For cat, it helps to visualize a startled
feline, back arched dramatically, claws gripping the earth.

Transition to movement

From the typically fairly static position of the body for breath
work at the start of a yoga session, it is usual to gently warm up
– especially the spine – before coming to more dynamic flows
and challenging poses. Cat-cow also provides a practical route
from your seated position to standing at the top of the mat,
ready for sun salutations.

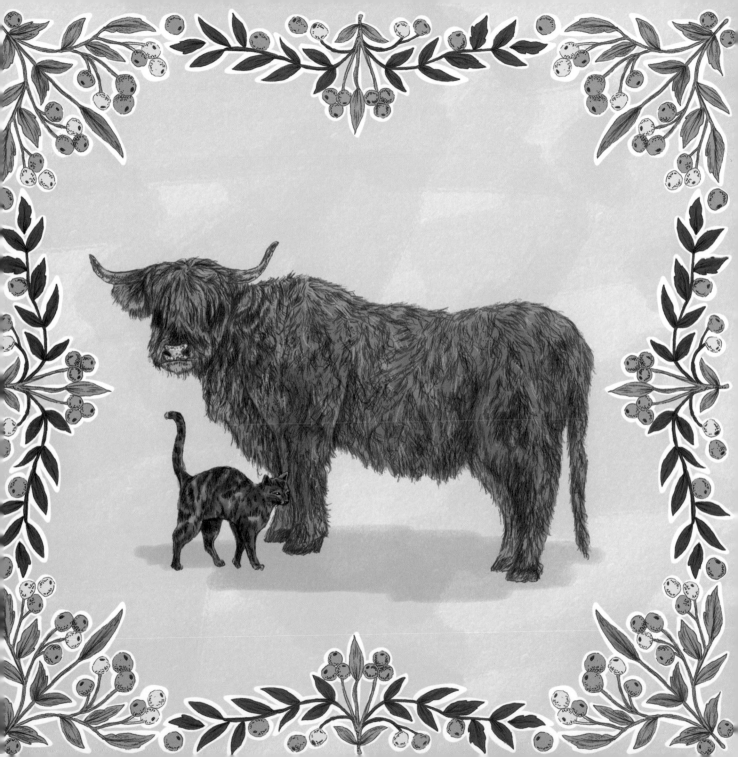

Cat-cow Pose Step by step

This two-pose flow (*vinyasa*) appears at the start of most yoga classes, forming the perfect transition from seated meditation and breathing practice to more dynamic or challenging poses and flows. This combination of poses will help you to practise the synchronization of movement and breath.

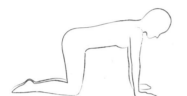

1 Make your way to all fours, with hands underneath the shoulders, knees underneath hips and neck in line with the rest of your spine. Spread the fingers and press down firmly through all four sides of the hands.

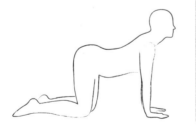

2 On an inhalation, drop the tummy, at the same time allowing the pointy sit bones in the bottom to move upwards. The gaze is straight ahead.

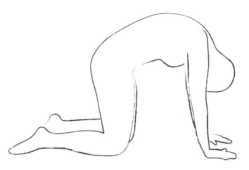

3 Exhale and draw the tummy inwards so that the belly button moves back towards the spine. Arch the upper back, allowing the head to drop towards the earth.

4 Flow back and forth between these two poses several more times, trying to synchronize cow to the length of your inhalation and cat to the duration of your exhalation.

5 Once you have established this flow you can make the movements even more fluid and intuitive, working into any nooks and crannies of the body that might feel they need more of a stretch or toning. You can also add a lift to the pelvic floor at the end of the exhalation to deepen the pose.

6 Come back to a neutral position on all fours.

Cobra

bhujangasana

Picture a snake's slithering forward movement when performing this pose, encouraging the work to be in the back muscles rather than craning the neck or using the strength of your arms to push up higher. Cobra pose is great for building this strength in the back muscles and stabilizing the spine. It acts as a lovely stretch for the front body, shoulders and lungs.

Back-bending poses can help access one's courage, owing to the bravery required to move without being able to see where you're going. Cobras can be used to symbolize rebirth, due to the shedding of their skin. Imagine sloughing off anything you would like to leave behind you as you practise this *asana*.

Sun salutations (*surya namaskar*)

Sun salutations work as a complete warm-up for the whole body, and depending on the speed and number of rounds, are more of a cardiovascular workout than much of standard yoga practice. The name originates with the Sanskrit word '*surya*' meaning 'sun' or the Hindu sun god. '*Namaskar*' means to greet or salute.

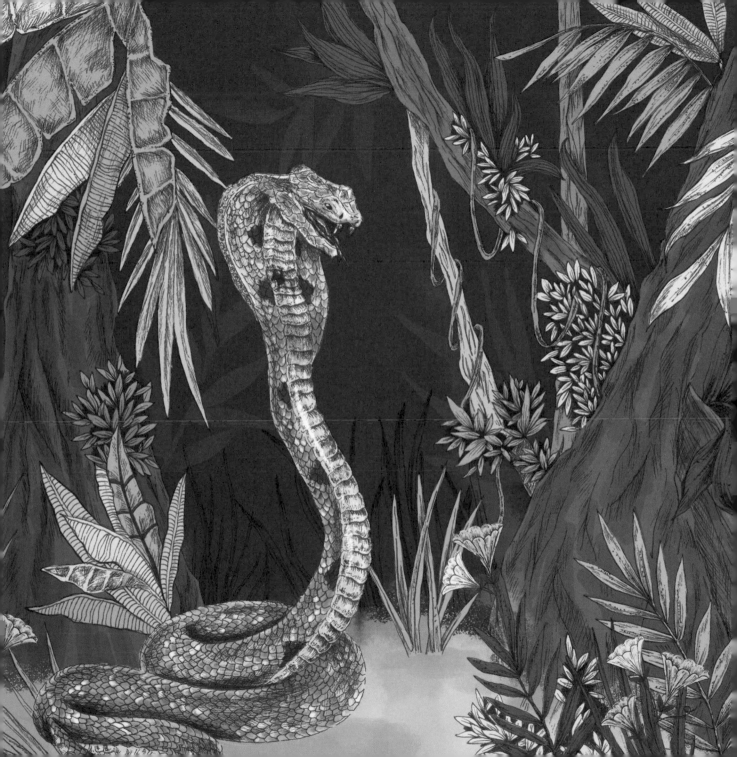

Cobra Pose Step by step

Cobra pose is a classic back bend, perfect for all levels of yoga experience, as it is possible to practise it very gently or as a stronger posture. It is performed in most versions of sun salutations, acting as the ideal way to gently warm up the back and build up to stronger back bends.

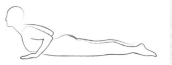

1 From a position lying on your front with your face down, bring your fingertips under your shoulders, your elbows drawing in. You can also come into cobra pose directly from lowering your knees, chest and chin to the floor in your sun salutations (see p 38–41).

2 Inhale, using only the muscles of the back to begin with, and lift the upper body off the ground. Keep the lower body pressing firmly into the ground. To ensure you are only using the back muscles, try floating the hands off the floor and see if you can maintain your position.

3 Exhale, lower back down.

4 Inhale, repeat but this time you can put a little
   pressure into the hands to lift up higher. Keep the
   muscles of the lower belly engaged, the elbows bent
   and drawing in, and the shoulders moving away from
   the ears. Make sure the pubic bone stays connected
   with the ground at all times.

5 When you're ready, come back to the ground on an
   exhalation. Repeat one more time.

Not quite ready for cobra pose?

Practise a gentler, more supported back bend with sphinx pose
(*salamba bhujangasana*).

Downward-facing Dog
adho mukha svanasana

Often one of the first poses people think of when considering
a modern physical yoga practice, downward-facing dog is the
ultimate stretch for the back body. However, it is also strengthening
for the arms and legs, meaning it can be a little tiring for new yoga
practitioners. This pose is the lynchpin of sun salutations, usually
being held for at least five breaths, which can offer a moment
of rest in the middle of the flow for experienced yogis.

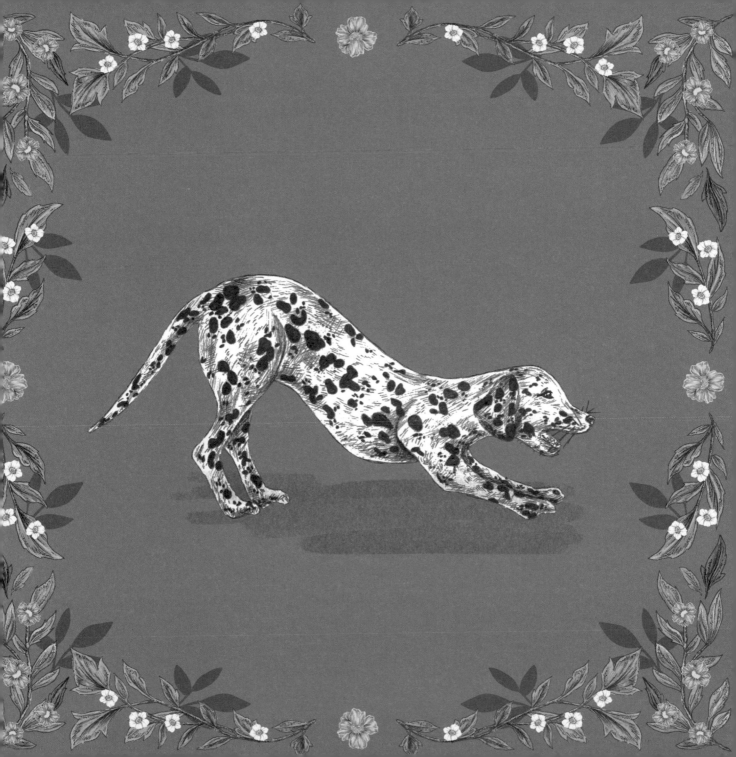

Downward-facing Dog Pose Step by step

There are many variations of the pose, which allow you
to achieve different benefits from it or to modify
it to suit your body's specific requirements.

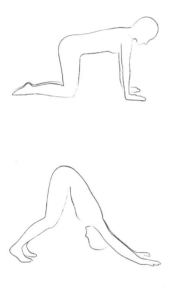

1 Come to all fours with the hands underneath the shoulders or just forward of them, knees underneath hips. Spread the fingers and press down firmly through all four sides of the hands. (You can also flow straight into downward dog from cobra or upward dog poses as part of your sun salutations – see p 38–41)

2 Tuck the toes under and, on an exhalation, push into the hands and lift the hips high.

3 If you have tighter hamstrings, you can keep the knees bent, gradually softening into the backs of the legs. Make sure not to lock the knees even if the legs are straight.

4 The heels will move towards the ground, but don't worry if they're still high.

5 Lengthen through the whole spine, gently drawing the belly button back towards it.

6 Shrug your shoulders away from the ears and flatten your shoulder blades across the back. Keep your neck in line with the rest of your spine. Do not raise your head. Your gaze should be focused on your feet.

7 Stay here for at least five breaths, if possible. To come out, either lower to all fours or continue with your sun salutations.

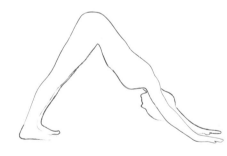

Not quite ready for or need a rest from downward dog pose?

Come back to all fours or rest in child's pose (*balasana*) – see p 80 for a reminder of how to come into this pose.

Upward-facing Dog
urdhva mukha svanasana

This pose is a counter to downward-facing dog (*adho mukha svanasana*), stretching the front body as the latter stretches the back. It is easy to picture a dog stretching in either upward- or downward-facing positions, really relishing the motion as it gets up refreshed from a nap. Upward-facing dog is also an alternative to cobra pose and can be performed in its place in your sun salutations, once you've sufficiently warmed up the back.

Dogs are often associated with loyalty, faithfulness and protection. In a similar way, upward and downward dog poses will be at the core of your yoga practice, always there to return to for a sense of home.

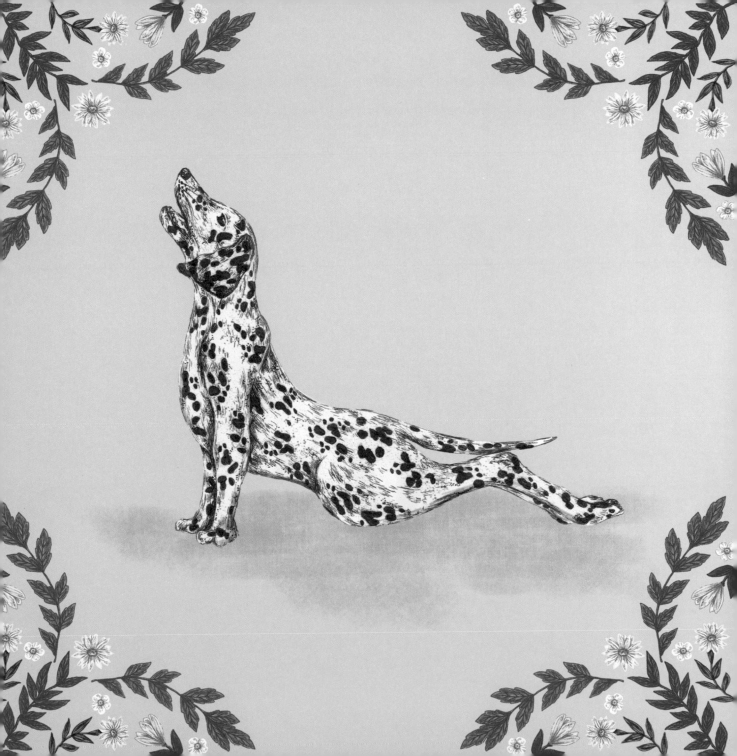

Upward-facing Dog Pose Step by step

Like cobra pose, upward-facing dog is strengthening for
the spine and a stretch for the front body, but it also builds
strength in the arms and wrists.

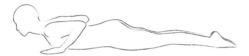

1 If the back is warmed up and injury free, from cobra pose
   on an inhalation you can walk the hands back a few inches
   towards the hips, straightening the arms. (You can also
   flow straight into upward dog from yoga reverse press-up,
   chaturanga dandasana. See sun salutations p 38–41.)

2 This will lift the legs off the floor, but make sure you keep
   the tops of the feet pressing firmly into the ground.

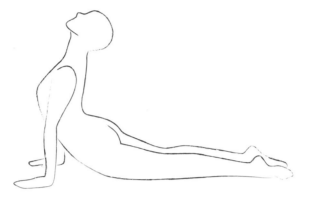

3 Drop the shoulders away from the ears and lift the upper chest without letting the ribs flare out. Keep some engagement in the lower belly muscles.

4 To come out, either lower to the floor or push back to downward-facing dog on an exhalation.

Sun Salutations (*surya namaskar*)
Step by step

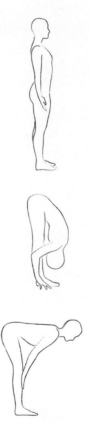

1 Stand in mountain pose (*tadasana*) at the top of your mat, feet rooted into the ground, spine straight, visualizing an invisible cord lifting you up through the top of your head. Eyes can be open or closed. Inhale. Exhale and bring your hands to your heart in prayer position.

2 Inhale, sweeping the arms up over the head. Exhale, taking the arms wide, coming all the way forward and down into a standing forward fold (*uttanasana*). Bend the knees as much as you need to in order to bring the fingertips in line with the tops of the toes.

3 Inhale, bring the hands to the shins or thighs in half-forward fold, so you have a flat back. Exhale, fold back down.

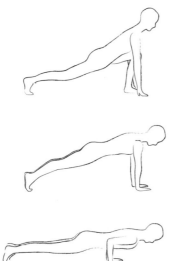

4 Inhale, step the right foot to the back of the mat.

5 Planting the hands, retaining the breath, step the left foot back to meet the right in a plank pose (*kumbhakasana*).

6 Exhale, move the knees, chin and chest down to the floor. Alternatively, bend the elbows, keeping them tucked in, and lower the body to the floor in a strong, straight line (*chaturanga dandasana*).

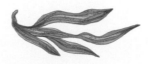

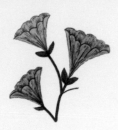

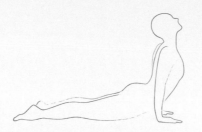

7 Inhale, sliding forward into cobra pose (*bhujangasana*) or upward-facing dog (*urdhva mukha svanasana*) if your lower back is strong and warmed up.

8 Exhale, pushing up and back into downward-facing dog (*adho mukha svanasana*). Take five nice long breaths here.

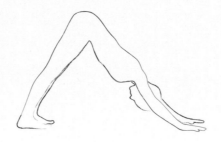

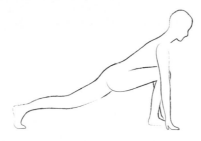

9 On your next inhalation, step the right foot forward between the hands.

10 Exhale, step the left foot forward to meet it.

11 Inhale, sweeping the arms wide, coming all the way up to stand in mountain pose.

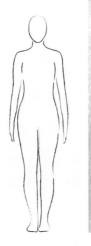

12 Exhale, bringing the hands back to prayer position at the heart. This is one round of sun salutations. Repeat, stepping the left foot back first. To warm up thoroughly, practise at least four rounds.

Horse

utkata konasana

This strong standing posture is also sometimes called goddess pose, so you can choose which energy you'd like to channel when practising. The name refers to the wide-legged, bent-knee stance, reminiscent of the position one assumes when riding a horse. The pose also appears in Asian martial arts, being a neutral but powerful position between strikes.

Horses are often used to symbolize freedom, due to the feeling riders experience and their association with travel. If a sense of freedom is elusive in this pose, you might like to add a gentle rocking motion.

Standing sequence

Once you've warmed up your whole body with some sun salutations, you can move on to a standing sequence. Such poses are a good opportunity to build heat in the body and get the heart rate going. They are also grounding and strengthening for the lower body in particular.

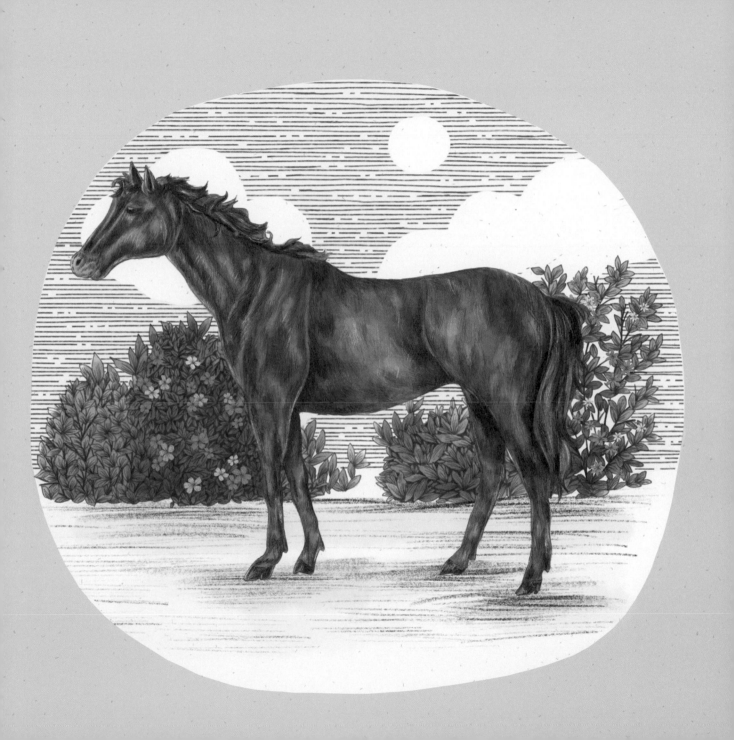

Horse Pose Step by step

Horse pose is suitable for all levels of yoga experience, because it can be practised more or less intensely. It works to both stretch and lengthen the lower body, and to open into the hips.

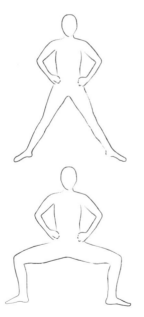

1 Step the feet a big stride apart, toes turning out.

2 On an exhalation, sink into the hips without sticking the bottom out.

3 The knees should be tracking straight over the feet, not rolling further in or outwards.

4 Keep the tailbone drawing downwards with the abdominal muscles engaged.

5 If you would like to intensify the pose, you can lift the arms overhead, palms facing upwards or towards each other. With time and practice, you may be able to bend the knees more deeply.

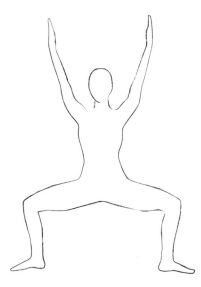

Standing Sequence
Step by step

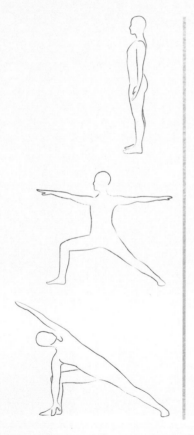

1 Come to stand in mountain pose (*tadasana*) at the top of your mat.

2 On an inhalation, step your left foot a big stride back. The right toes should be pointing straight forward, the left turning slightly out. Exhale and bend the right knee deeply, lifting the arms alongside the ears in warrior 1 (*virabhadrasana* 1). Keep the hips square and facing forward.

3 Inhale and open your arms and hips out to the left in warrior 2 (*virabhadrasana* 2). Stay here as you exhale.

4 Inhale, bringing the right forearm to the right thigh, left arm up and over your ear in extended side angle pose (*utthita parsvakonasana*). Stay here as you exhale. To deepen the pose, you can bring your right hand to the floor inside your right foot.

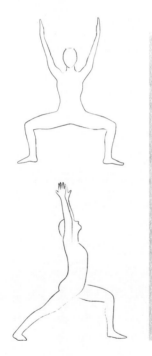

5 Inhale, windmilling the arms back up, turning the left toes out and the right toes in slightly. As you exhale, bend the knees, sinking the hips into horse pose. Lift the arms. Stay here for a few breaths.

6 Inhale, spinning on the ball of the right foot to turn to face the back of the mat, coming into warrior 1 on the second side. Repeat the rest of the sequence on this side.

7 Flow through the whole sequence twice more to build heat and strength.

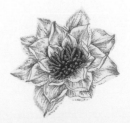

Eagle
garudasana

This challenging balancing pose requires focus and patience. In English, it is usually known simply as 'eagle', but the Sanskrit word derives from the name 'Garuda' – legendary king of the birds and sun bird in Hindu mythology, ridden by the god Vishnu. You might find it helpful to picture a powerful bird of prey perching with wings furled when practising eagle pose – or lean in to the challenge and visualize yourself in flight, navigating the winds and currents at the highest altitude.

Standing balances

Standing balances help you develop strength while finding focus and calm. Your ability to perform them may vary from day to day: practice helps, but emotions and hormones also play a part in their achievability. Key to all balancing postures is finding a steady, still focus point for your gaze ahead of you (your *drishti*). This gaze should be soft and can act as an anchor and means of drawing the awareness to the present moment .

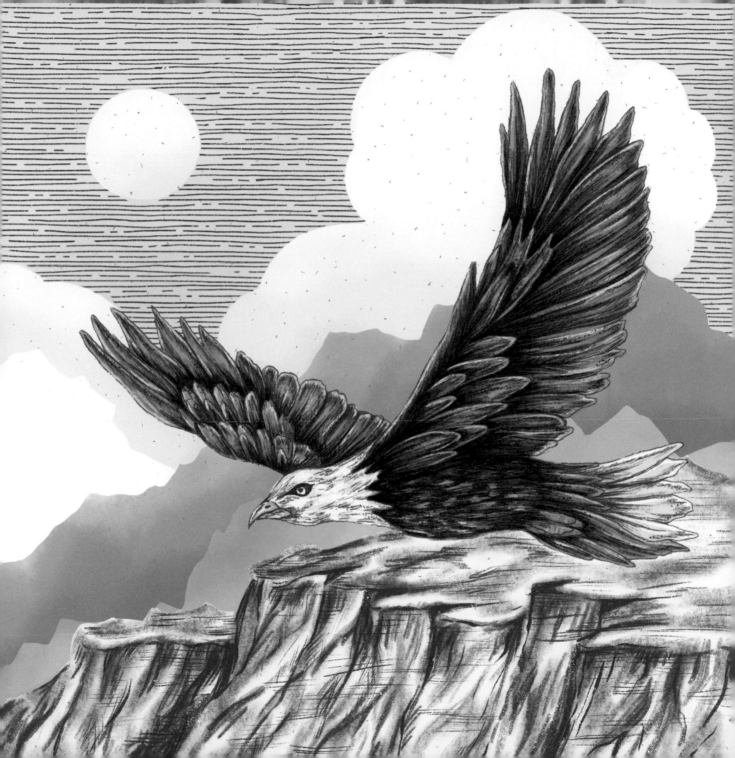

Eagle Pose Step by step

Eagle pose both stretches and strengthens the legs, and also stretches the upper back and shoulders. It is a good standing balance to practise after warming up the body and strengthening the muscles with sun salutations and a standing flow.

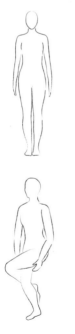

1 Come to stand in the middle of your mat. Find your steady gaze point (*drishti*) on the ground ahead.

2 Feel yourself rooted and grounded through both feet and legs, then put a little bend in the knees.

3 On an inhalation, lift the left knee and wrap the left thigh over the right, tucking the left toes behind the right calf if possible. Bring both knees back to the midline and sink deeper into the hips.

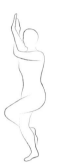

4 On your next inhalation, take the arms out at shoulder height. Bend the elbows and wrap the left arm under the right, forearms also folding around each other and, if possible, bringing the palms to touch.

5 Breathe deeply. Lift the elbows and move the hands away from the face. If you have a wobble, take a breath and then come back in.

6 Stay here for a few breaths, then come out slowly and with control, reversing the actions you took to come into the pose.

7 Repeat on the second side.

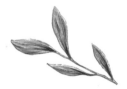

Not quite ready for eagle pose?

Practise finding your balance with tree pose (*vrksasana*).
Build strength in the thighs with chair pose (*utkatasana*).
Open into the shoulders with cow face pose (*gomukhasana*) – see p 64.

Half Lord of the Fishes
ardha matsyendrasana

This is perhaps the most famous of the yoga twists. The Sanskrit title for the pose comes from the name 'Matsyendra' – a saint and yogi in some Hindu and Buddhist traditions who is also credited with writing various early hatha yoga texts. Matsyendra is known as 'lord of the fishes', with legends differing as to whether this is because he was a fisherman, was swallowed by a fish or even was born as a fish!

You might like to picture a fish using its gills to breathe, as you breathe deeply into the back of the lungs.

Seated twists

Now make your way to the floor. Twisting poses bring a fresh supply of oxygenated blood rushing back into the areas of the body that have been constricted during the twist. They can stimulate the digestive system and improve flexibility in the spine, perfect for counteracting a lot of time spent at a desk and helping to improve posture.

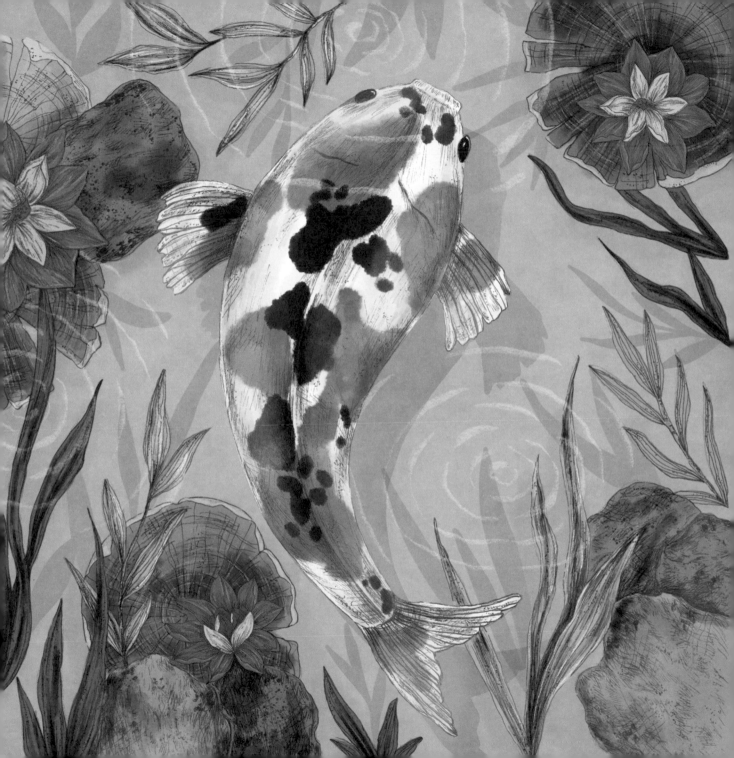

Half Lord of the Fishes Pose Step by step

When practising this pose, it might help to visualize your spine as a spiral staircase: each inhalation takes you up a step; each exhalation further round. While the arms are used, try to initiate the movement from the inner body, rather than using them to force yourself further into the pose.

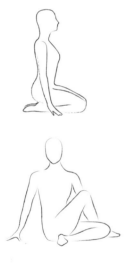

1 Come to kneel on your mat. Inhale and sit the bottom to the left of the feet. Step the right foot over the left thigh, the right knee pointing towards the sky.

2 On your next inhalation, raise the right arm up, creating space in the right side body, before taking the right hand to the ground behind you, flat on the floor with fingertips pointing away from you, as close to the sacrum (the flat bone at the base of your spine) as you can get it.

3 Inhale and raise the left arm, extending through the left side body. As you exhale, bend the left elbow and take it to the right side of the right knee or thigh. With the left hand, reach for the right foot. If you can't take hold of the foot, bend the left elbow and wrap it around the right knee instead.

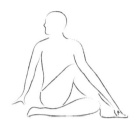

4 Now close your eyes and take your awareness inwards, visualizing the organs, muscles and spine in your abdominal region. Initiating the movement here, on your next inhalation, lengthen through the spine, exhale and twist to the right.

5 Keep moving in this way with the breath, aiming to move the belly button past the right thigh. If your neck is comfortable you can turn the head over the right shoulder. When you've reached your maximum twist, stay here and breathe. If you are experienced and flexible, you may find it possible to thread the left arm under the right thigh, the right arm round the back of the left waist, so they can meet and clasp. This is known as a yoga bind.

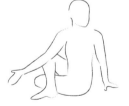

6 To come out, untwist with control, bringing the left arm behind you and the right arm inside the right knee to take a brief counter twist.

7 Come back to kneeling and then repeat on the second side.

Deer

Deer pose is a gentle posture from the yin yoga tradition. Yin integrates aspects of Chinese medicine with yoga *asana*, and works with longer, often supported, holds to access and release the deep connective tissue in the body. Because of its slow, unrushed style, yin can also help to deactivate the sympathetic nervous system (the fight or flight response), allowing secondary but important functions in the body such as digestion to kick in. However, this is not to say that yin is *easy*. Longer holds can bring their own challenges, both physical and psychological.

This posture's name is self-explanatory. While it is a gentle, still pose, you might like to visualize the powerful legs of a leaping stag or doe. Deer appear in world mythology in a range of ways, from incarnations of deities and royalty in disguise, to symbols of heroic quests. There is something majestic and magical about this pose, so enjoy these possibilities as you practise.

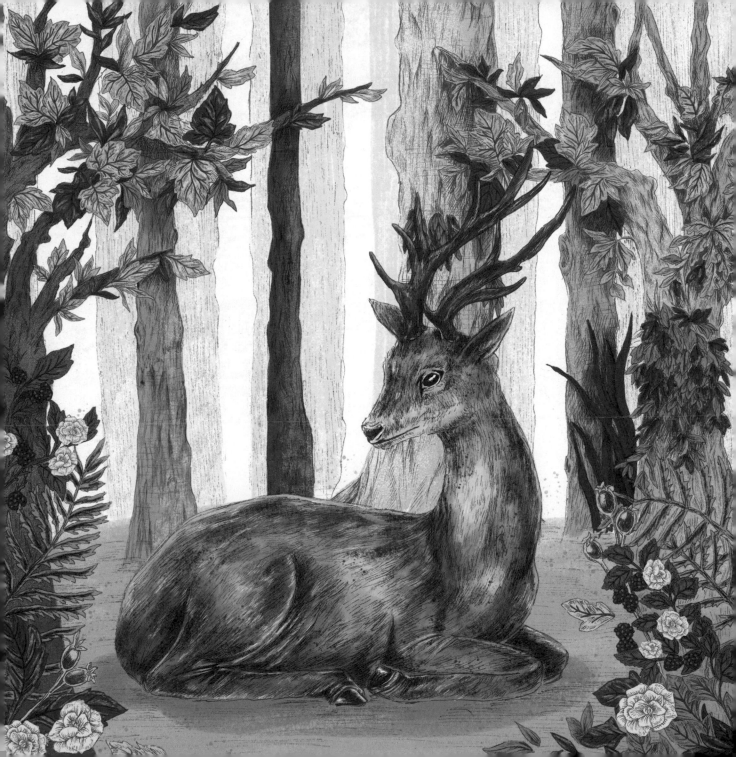

Deer Pose Step by step

Ideally, deer pose should be held for a few minutes on each side to access the benefits of a yin practice. However, beginners or those working with injuries or simply discomfort can hold for a shorter time. As well as the usual benefits of a twist, this pose also opens into the hips.

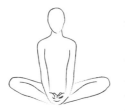

1 Come to sit with the soles of the feet together, knees opening outwards.

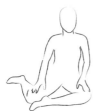

2 On an inhalation, take the right leg behind you. Both knees should now have a 90-degree angle, the left leg externally rotating and the right internally rotating, and both soles of the feet pointing towards the right side of the body. However, adjust the leg position to be at more acute angles if this does not feel comfortable.

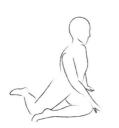

3 On your next inhalation, draw up tall through the spine and – again initiating the movement from the inner body – twist the upper body to the left as you exhale, bringing the hands to the floor outside the left thigh. The torso is now to the left of both legs.

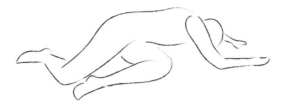

4 Stay here if this is enough. Otherwise, you can push into the hands to lift the left hip, move it slightly backward, then lower it and fold the upper body forward. You can use a pillow or bolster to support the upper body here.

5 Stay here and breathe.

6 When you're ready to come out, untwist and then repeat on the second side.

Butterfly
baddha konasana

This is a yin yoga variation of bound angle pose (*baddha konasana*). The name comes from the opening knees, which can be pictured as gently flapping butterfly wings. Butterflies have connotations with rebirth or reincarnation, and transformation, going as they do from one form to a completely different form as they metamorphose from a caterpillar to a butterfly. Be open to potential and seemingly miraculous change as you practise this pose, and who knows what might happen!

Hip-openers

Hip-opening poses are another good way of countering a sedentary lifestyle, as well as the effects of other dynamic forms of exercise. It is believed that our hips store a lot of emotional memory, which could explain why they are so often an area of tightness, and why many feelings can arise as we begin to work into this region. Practise these poses with patience and self-compassion.

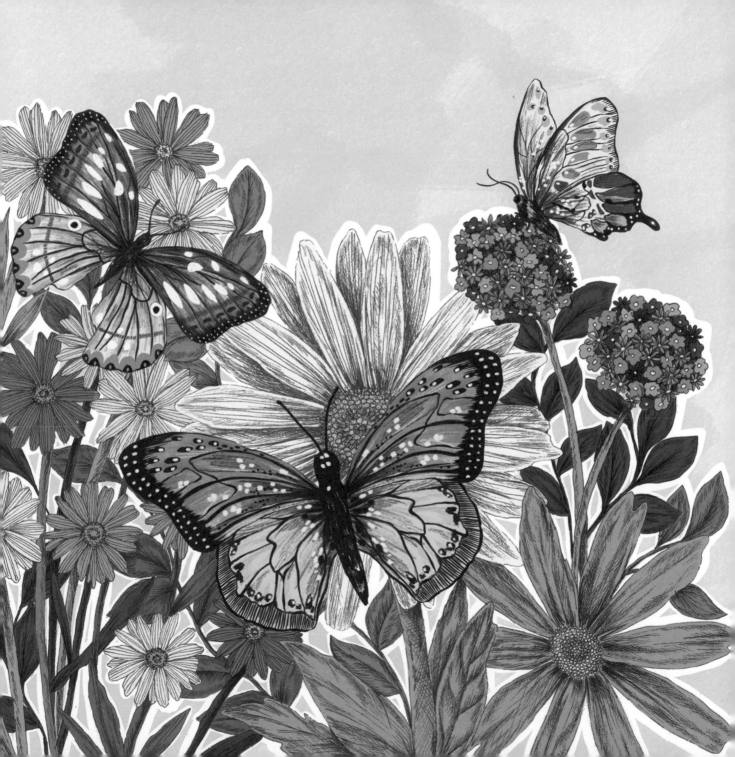

Butterfly Pose Step by step

This pose is a gentle and gradual way of opening into the hips and inner thighs, which can act as the perfect introduction to stronger hip-openers.

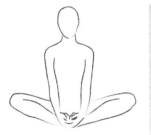

1 Come to sit on the ground with the soles of the feet together, hands cupped gently around the feet. The sit bones should be firmly in contact with the floor. If you are rounding in the lower back, it might help to sit on the edge of a yoga block or cushion, to allow you to lift up out of the hips and tilt the pelvis.

2 For bound angle pose you might move your hips towards your feet to intensify the stretch. However, for longer holds of yin, a more open posture is preferable – therefore, you may wish to move your hips further away from your feet.

3 Keeping the outside edges of the feet touching, open the inside edges outwards.

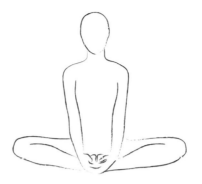

4 Draw up nice and tall and, as you exhale, soften the hips and gently squeeze the muscles of the outer thighs and glutes to allow the knees to drop lower.

5 Inhale to lengthen through the spine and release this effort, then exhale to softly squeeze again without forcing the knees downwards. Repeat at least once more.

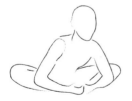

6 If you would like to go further, you can hinge the upper body forward on an exhalation, just to the point where you feel sensation but no pain. Then stay here and breathe.

7 To come out, cup your hands under your knees to carefully bring them back together.

Cow Face
gomukhasana

It is believed that the name comes from the shape we make in the pose – the folded and stacked legs are the cow's mouth, the raised elbow represents one lifted ear – and it is described in the text of the *Hatha Yoga Pradipika*, which is over 500 years old.

While this pose can be challenging for many, perhaps you might find it helpful to imagine the calm and placid nature of a cow, allowing yourself to soften and release into it rather than straining or struggling. Cows are often associated with the nurturing, caring side of nature. Treat this pose as an opportunity for self-nurture and work with kindness towards yourself.

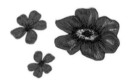

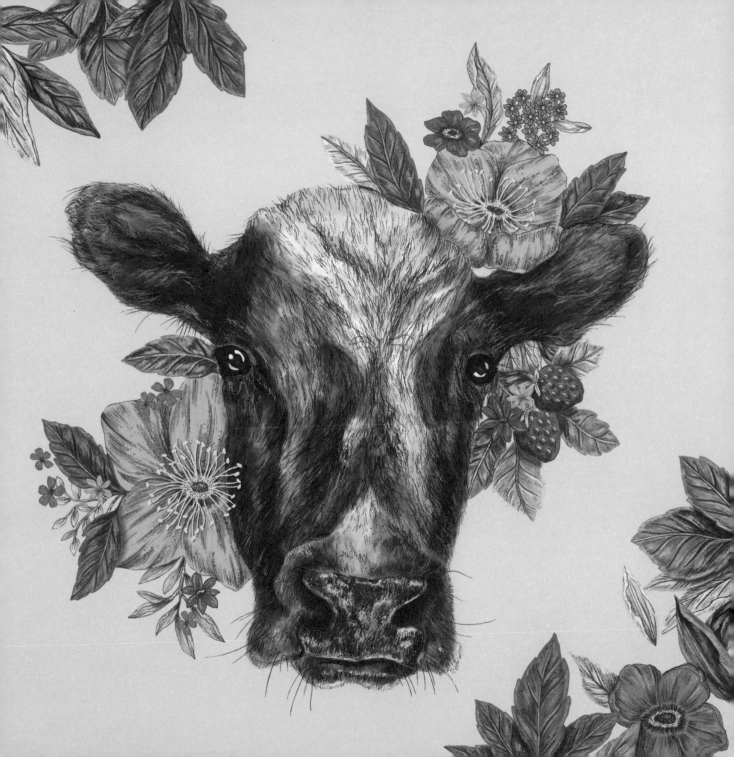

Cow Face Pose Step by step

This stronger hip-opening posture also acts as a big stretch for the side body and shoulders – but it's possible to modify or even use a different arm position if tight shoulders are preventing you from performing it.

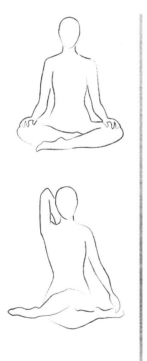

1 Come to sit in a cross-legged position with the left leg in front. Gently move the left knee towards the midline, taking the left foot to the outside of the right hip.

2 Stack the right knee underneath the left, the right foot coming to the outside of the left hip. If you have tighter hips you might find that the knees are very far apart, but don't worry about this. Support the body as required with folded blankets, blocks or cushions, and breathe into any areas of tightness.

3 On an inhalation, take the right arm up alongside the right ear, then bend the elbow, dropping the right hand between the two shoulder blades. You can use your left hand on the right elbow to gently guide the right hand a little further down the back.

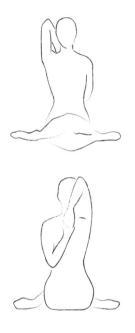

4 Now take the left arm out to the side, bend the elbow, take the back of the left hand to the spine and swim it up between the shoulder blades. If the fingers reach, you can clasp them. Otherwise, hold onto your clothing, a yoga strap or a scarf.

5 Notice if the head is being knocked forward by the arms; if so, try to bring it back into alignment with the spine.

6 Breathe deeply and slowly in the pose. Stay here if this is enough or, to intensify the hip stretch, hinge forward to the point of strong sensation (but not pain).

7 When you are ready, carefully come out and repeat on the second side.

Not quite ready for cow face pose?

Butterfly (see p 60) and yoga squat (*malasana*) act as good warm-ups for the hips. Practise kneeling thread-the-needle to open into the shoulders.

Lizard

utthan pristhasana

This is another pose whose English name needs little explanation once you've seen or performed it yourself. The Sanskrit name actually translates as 'page-stretching pose', which provides a different visual cue as you imagine pulling the mat apart between your feet. It can form part of a standing flow sequence (*vinyasa*), or be practised in isolation, and it is possible to both modify and build on it.

Lizards are stealthy and patient hunters, usually preferring to wait for an opportune moment rather than launch a proactive attack. So, too, you will find patience very helpful when practising this posture, and the best way to reap the benefits of it.

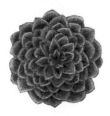

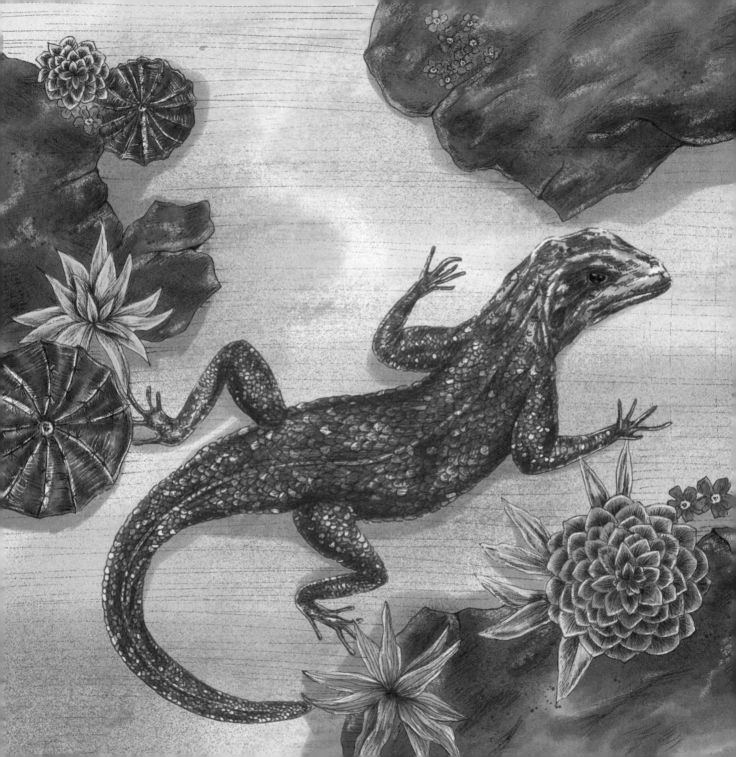

Lizard Pose Step by step

As well as being a hip-opener, lizard lunge is a good way
of both stretching and strengthening the groin and
the hamstring and quadriceps muscles in the legs.

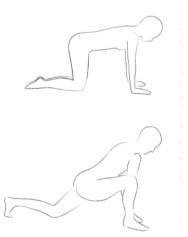

1 Come to all fours with the hands underneath the
shoulders, knees underneath the hips.

2 Step the right foot forward to the outside of the
right hand, toes lining up with fingertips, right
knee over right ankle. If your hips are tighter or
not warmed up yet, you might like to heel-toe the
right foot further out to the right, and you can
also turn the toes out to the right to help create
more space.

3 You can keep the left knee on the floor or tuck
the back toes under and lift it now to intensify
the work.

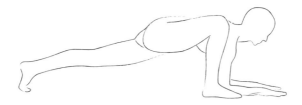

4 On an exhalation, lower onto the forearms. You can
use a block to bring the floor closer, or stay on the hands
if this feels strong enough.

5 Flatten the shoulder blades and broaden through
the collarbones.

6 Stay here and breathe. You can add a gentle rocking
motion if that brings greater ease to the pose.

7 To come out, make your way back to all fours, then
repeat on the second side.

Not quite ready for lizard pose?

Stretch and strengthen the hips and legs in crescent pose
(*anjaneyasana*) or high lunge.

Swan & One-legged King Pigeon
eka pada rajakapotasana

Swan is also sometimes known as 'sleeping swan', because you fold forward over the front leg – but don't forget that while swans look calm and elegant on the surface of the water, a lot of work is going on out of view! King pigeon involves puffing the chest forward like its avian namesake. Both require externally rotating the front leg and hip, and stretching the hip flexors. You can choose which option feels more beneficial to you today, or practise both!

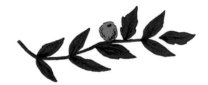

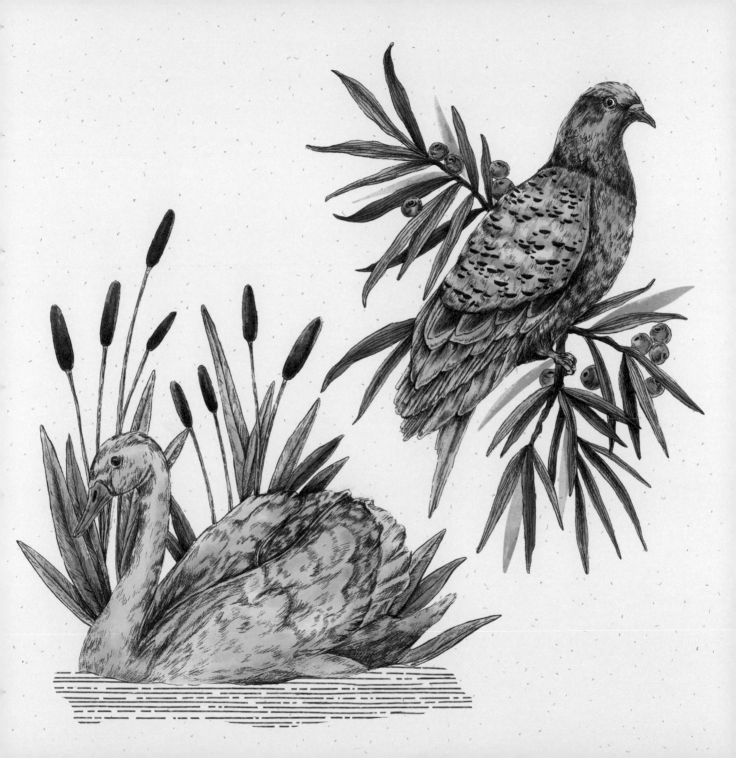

Swan Pose Step by step

These two poses are different variations of each other: swan is a yin-style restorative pose, the more relaxed of the two.

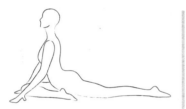

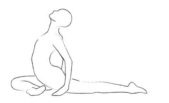

1 From all fours or downward-facing dog, bring the right knee forward, next to the right wrist, lowering the right shin onto the floor.

2 Push into the hands to lift the hips off the ground and draw the pelvis level before lowering back to the floor.

3 To create more space you can tuck the back toes under and move the left knee backward. Your left leg should extend straight out from the hip.

4 Inhale to lengthen through the spine, exhale to fold forward. You can use a pillow or bolster to support yourself if necessary. Come to a point at which you have sensation and stretch but not pain – this might mean staying up on the hands or folding fully forward, depending on your body and the day.

5 Stay here and breathe for a couple of minutes.

6 To come out, push back up to all fours or downward dog and repeat on the other side, bringing your left knee to the left wrist.

Not quite ready for swan?

Prime the hips by practising three-legged dog.

One-legged King Pigeon Pose
Step by step

King pigeon is a stronger and more dynamic version of the pose,
with back-bending and quadriceps-stretching options.

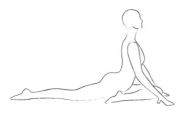

1 From all fours or downward-facing dog, bring the left knee forward, next to the left wrist, lowering the left shin onto the floor. To intensify the stretch, gently guide the shin towards being parallel with the front edge of your mat.

2 Push into the hands to lift the hips off the ground and draw the pelvis level before lowering back to the floor.

3 To create more space, you can tuck the back toes under and move the right knee backward. Your right leg should extend straight out from the hip.

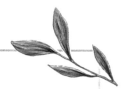

4 Keeping the tailbone long and heavy, puff the chest out, bringing the hands to the hips or extending them alongside the ears. Feel the back muscles engage and draw the lower belly in to support them.

5 If your neck feels comfortable, you can carefully drop the head back to look up, maybe arching into the upper back.

6 Stay here for a few breaths.

7 When you're ready to come out, make your way back to all fours or downward dog and repeat on the other side.

Want to take your one-legged king pigeon pose further?

Try bending the back knee and reaching for the inside edge of the back foot with the hand on the same side – and on the opposite side for a different challenge. You can also stand the front foot on the floor and bend the back knee for another variation of the pose.

Frog

adho mukha mandukasana

There are a number of yoga poses named 'frog', but, for our purposes, we are going to focus on the one whose Sanskrit name translates as 'downward-facing frog' – a strong hip-opener that the previous poses will have helped you warm up for. There is no way to muscle into this pose if your body is not ready for it!

Feel free to support and cushion yourself in this pose, to allow yourself to stay in it for a few moments at least. You might like to double up the mat or put a blanket under the knees, or have a cushion or bolster to prop up the arms and bring the floor closer. Picture a frog's supple legs moving it through water or on land to bring a sense of fluidity and flexibility, even while staying still in the pose.

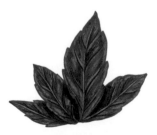

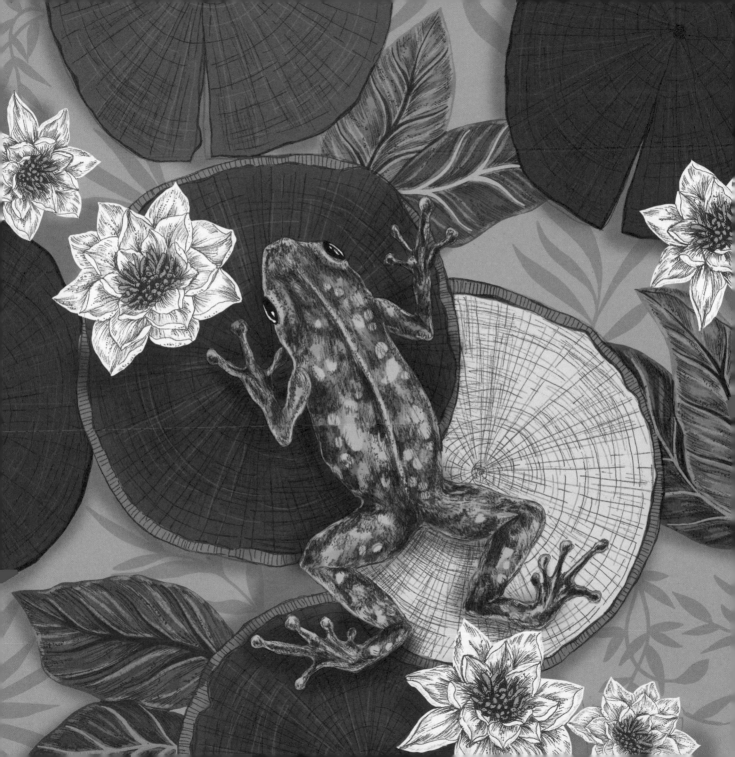

Frog Pose Step by step

Unless you have naturally very mobile hips, this pose will be a challenge
and will require especial patience, and gentle softening and releasing.

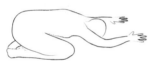

1 Come to a wide-legged child's pose (*balasana*)
variation: big toes touching, knees as wide as
the mat, arms and upper body reaching forward
on the ground.

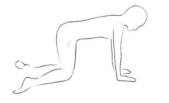

2 Come up onto the forearms or hands. Bring the
ankles in line with the knees, feet turning outwards.

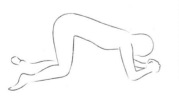

3 If you are up on the hands, try to lower the
forearms back to the floor, hands clasped.

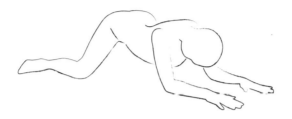

4 On an exhalation, move the hips backward until you can feel a strong stretch (but no pain) in the hips and inner thighs.

5 Stay here and breathe, allowing the hips to descend towards the floor. With time, you might feel able to take your knees wider, and the upper body and hips may move closer towards the ground.

6 To come out, gradually make your way back onto all fours. Rest in child's pose with the knees together.

Heron
krounchasana

Heron pose is a strong hamstring stretch that should not be attempted without warming up thoroughly beforehand, but which may nevertheless continue to be a challenge for those with tighter hamstrings. It also stretches the calf of the extended leg and the quadriceps of the bent leg.

Herons are known for being quiet, steady and patient, and are associated with this stillness, peace and determination. Picture a heron's one long and elegant leg plunging through water, the other tucked underneath it as it waits and watches, to bring the same sense of grace to this pose.

Forward folds

These poses are brilliant for balancing out strengthening work – not just in yoga but also in other dynamic forms of exercise. Seated forward folds are also a very good place to practise using your breath to soften and release, to keep bringing the attention back to the present moment – over-efforting will not get you far in these poses!

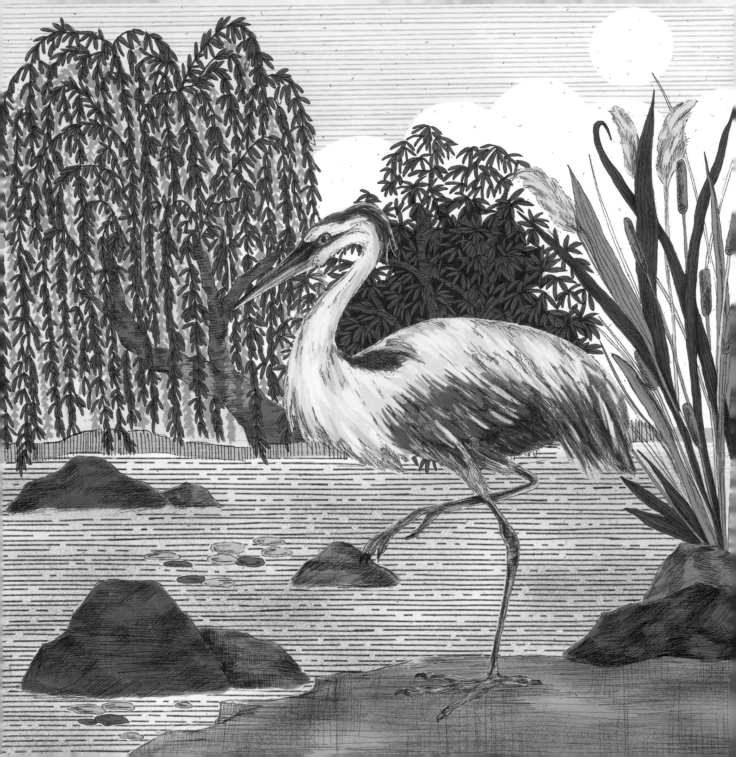

Heron Pose Step by step

This pose is great for stretching the whole back body,
as well as turning the awareness inwards.

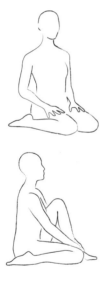

1 Come to sit in hero pose (*virasana*), kneeling with the knees together, bottom nestled between the feet, toes untucked. If this is already very challenging – and if the bottom doesn't reach the floor – you can put a block, bolster or folded blanket between the feet.

2 Bring the left leg in front of you, knee bent and left foot just in front of the left sitting bone.

3 Reach inside the left leg with the right arm, taking hold of the inside edge of the left foot.

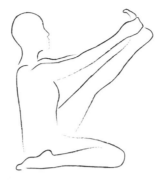

4 Now, reach outside the left leg with the left arm, taking hold of the outside edge of the left foot.

5 On an inhalation, lean back slightly, keeping both the spine and the front body long.

6 Exhale to lift the left leg towards a 45-degree angle. Stay here and breathe.

7 When you're ready to come out, carefully lower the left leg to the floor, fold it in and repeat with the right leg.

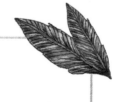

Not quite ready for heron pose?

Stretch the hamstrings in seated forward fold (*paschimottanasana*). Stretch the thighs in reclining hero pose (*supta virasana*).

Tortoise
kurmasana

One of the first things that comes to mind when thinking about a tortoise is a certain inwardness, a sheltering within one's shell: in other words, exactly what I referred to earlier in terms of the psychological and emotional experience of forward folds. This pose benefits from you having already stretched into the back, hips and backs of legs, so if you are working through the book chronologically, now is the perfect time to practise it.

Tortoises are known for living for a very long time, and also for being skilled at self-protection – two features that may not be unrelated! They are also associated with wisdom. Channel the no-rushing attitude of a tortoise, allow your back to round like your protective shell and breathe into the challenge.

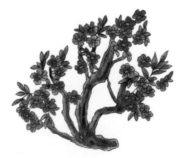

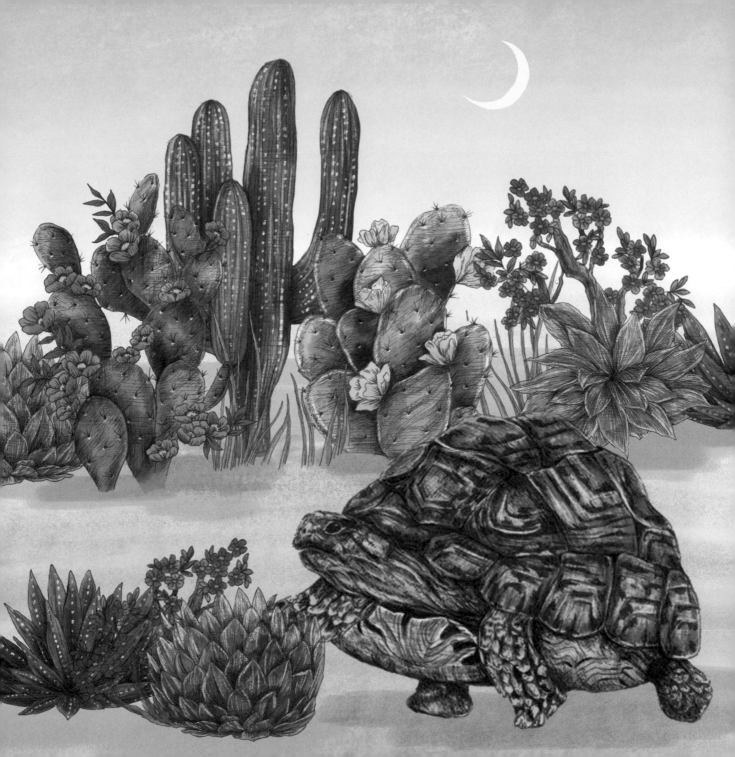

Tortoise Pose Step by step

As this is a strong back-body stretch, those with tighter hamstrings may find it a challenge regardless of how warmed up or experienced they are.

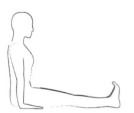

1 Come to sit in staff pose (*dandasana*): sitting bones firmly in contact with the ground, legs outstretched and together, feet flexed, spine upright and arms alongside the upper body, palms on the floor next to the hips.

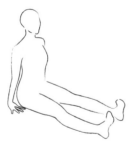

2 Inhale, taking the feet wider than shoulder-distance apart.

3 Bending your knees slightly, one at a time, thread your right arm under the right thigh, left arm under left thigh, palms down.

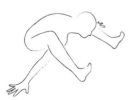

4 Lengthen through the spine on an inhalation, and – if you have room to go further – fold forward on your exhalation. You can use a bolster or cushion to bring the floor closer.

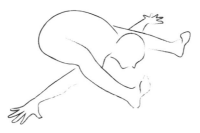

5 Use your breath to scan the body. If this pose is challenging, the chances are you will notice places of tension and holding. Can you direct your breath to these places to soften and release? Picture again that tortoise, safe and comfortable in its shell, prepared to wait for what it needs. Breathe that same sense of ease into your body.

6 To come out, unthread the arms, take the hands behind the knees and draw the legs into the body.

Not quite ready for tortoise pose?

Stretch the hamstrings and hips in wide-legged forward fold (*prasarita padottanasana*). Use gravity to assist your hamstring stretch in standing forward fold (*uttanasana*).

Monkey
hanumanasana

Known throughout Western culture and in gymnastics as the forward splits, this pose is synonymous with preternatural flexibility, and many may feel it is outside the realms of possibility for them. However, there are ways of working towards this posture that accrue many of the benefits of the full pose, even if that itself proves elusive.

Hanuman is the Hindu monkey god, and the pose is said to commemorate his athletic leap to the island of Sri Lanka to rescue Sita in the ancient text, the *Ramayana*. Perhaps visualizing this leap of faith – the impossible somehow becoming possible – will help in practising this challenging pose. Monkeys are known for being intelligent but are also often linked with ideas of playfulness and fun. Cultivating all these characteristics will only serve you in this posture.

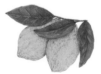

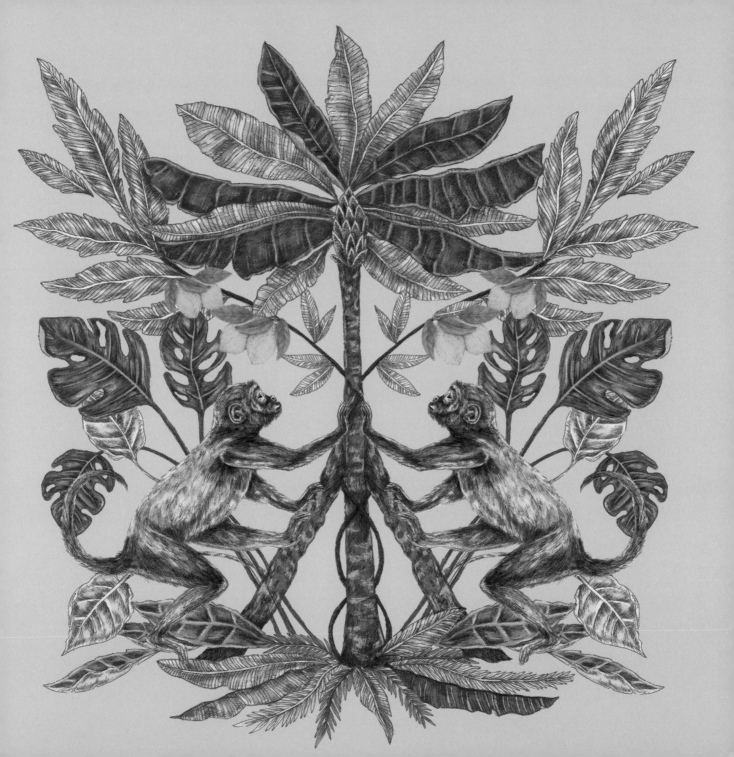

Monkey Pose Step by step

While the obvious stretch in this pose happens in the hamstrings,
monkey pose also targets flexibility in the thighs and groin.

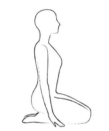

1 Come to a kneeling position on the floor and then extend your right leg out in front of you.

2 Bring the hands to the floor or to blocks to support yourself as you lift up and slide the left leg backward, the top of the leg facing towards the ground.

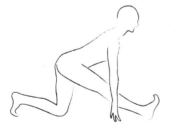

3 Push into the hands to draw your inner thighs towards each other, then tuck the left toes under. Flex the right foot.

4 Gradually, working with the breath, inch the right heel forward and the left foot backward until you come to your comfortable edge of sensation. Stay here and breathe. As you continue to breathe and soften, and particularly with time and practice, you might find it possible to inch the feet slightly further apart, the legs closer to being straight.

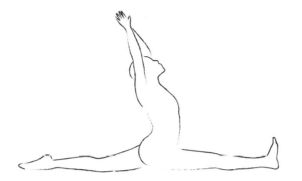

5 If you can come into full monkey pose, you might like to bring the hands to the heart in prayer position, or the arms overhead, palms facing, which works the back muscles.

6 To come out, bring the hands back to the floor or blocks to support yourself as you move very gradually to bring the legs back towards each other.

7 Repeat on the second side.

Not quite ready for monkey pose?

Work on hamstring and hip flexibility in runner's lunge (*ardha hanumanasana*) or pyramid pose (*parsvottanasana*).

Locust

salabhasana

While still fitting firmly in the category of back bends, locust pose is a good place to practise and warm up for them. It works all the muscles of the back body in a gentle way, helping to bring strength and support to this area, while also opening the front body. As these muscles become stronger, you might find it possible to move into a fuller version of the pose, knees bending and feet moving towards the head. Whatever level you practise it to, picture the elegance and agility of the eponymous creatures, imagining the powerful leaps you could be capable of.

Backward bends

Self-evidently the opposite of forward bends, backward bends have a showier, more extroverted side than their inward-facing counterparts. They can also be associated with heart-opening, bravery or, conversely, bringing up feelings of vulnerability in the very nature of moving the body into a space you can't see.

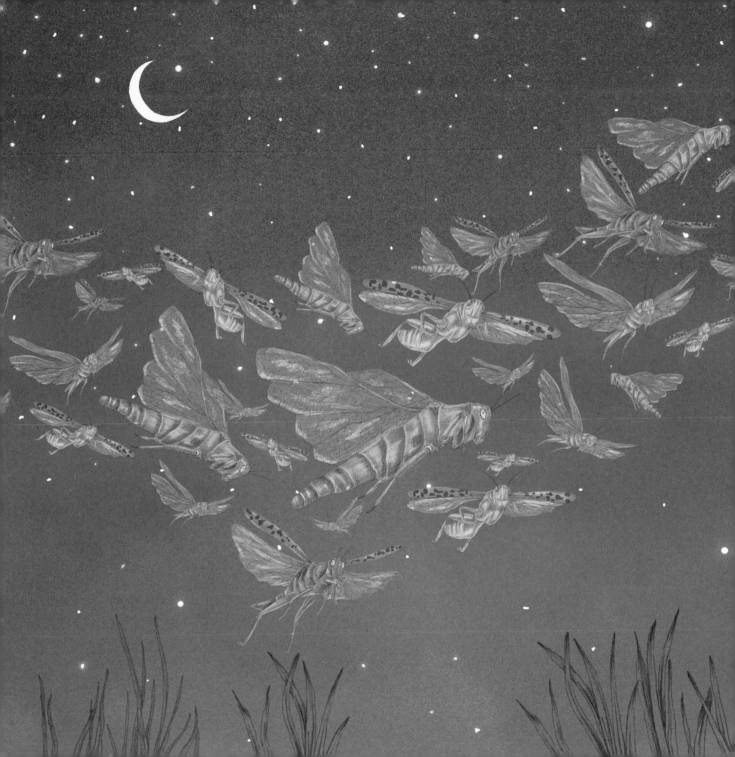

Locust Pose Step by step

Locust pose works to open into the front body while
constricting and contracting in the back body.

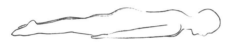

1 Come to lie on your front with your face down,
arms alongside the body, palms face down
on the mat.

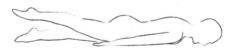

2 First, it helps to move all the different muscles
of the back body in isolation. Begin, on an
inhalation, by peeling only the right leg off
the floor, extending from big toe all the way
to hip. Lower on the exhalation. Repeat this
with the left leg.

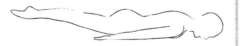

3 Now, lift both legs together, keeping the upper
body pressing into the ground.

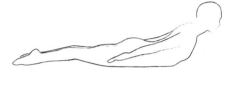

4 Next, lift only the upper body, feeling the muscles of the back engage, keeping the neck long. The legs lie heavy on the ground.

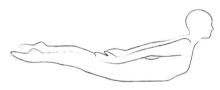

5 On your next inhalation, lift the legs and upper body at the same time, arms alongside the body. Lower to the floor on the exhalation.

6 Repeat, this time with the option of bringing the arms alongside the ears, which might allow you to lift a little higher.

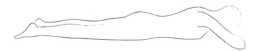

7 Lower on an exhalation, bringing the big toes to touch, heels falling apart. Make a pillow with your hands and turn your face to one side, resting against them.

Seal
bhujangasana variation

This pose is an extension of cobra or sphinx poses, the latter providing the entry route to this posture. As such, it's a more intense back bend, compressing into the lower back and stimulating these muscles, as well as the kidneys and the adrenal glands. In addition to it being a back bend and a chest opener, practising this pose can strengthen the arms.

Picture a seal basking on a rock by the sea, fin-shaped feet outstretched, preparing to plunge through the water with speed and grace. Some species of seal are able to hold their breath beneath the water for up to two hours at a time, conserving oxygen by slowing their heart rate. Cultivate that same sense of ease and pacing oneself when practising this pose.

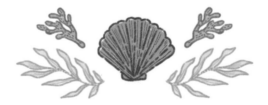

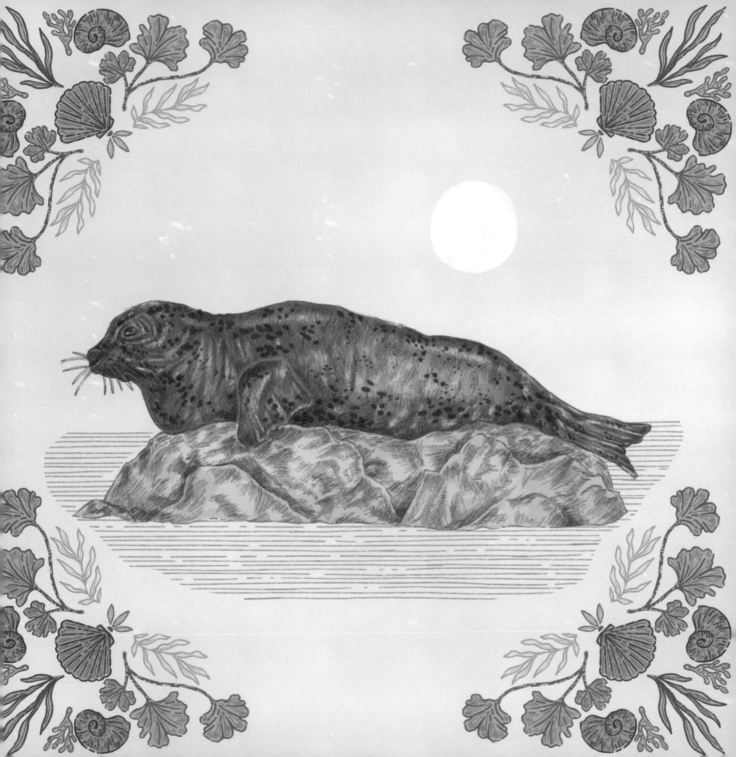

Seal Pose Step by step

Seal pose can be practised as part of a yin yoga session,
and, if holding for longer, you may like to support
the upper body with a bolster or cushion.

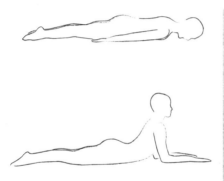

1 Come to lie face down on the ground.

2 Bring the elbows directly underneath the shoulders,
the forearms parallel, lifting up into sphinx
pose (*salamba bhujangasana*). Broaden through
the collarbones and draw the muscles of the
lower belly inwards to protect the lower back.

3 Stay here if this is a strong enough back bend.
Otherwise, rotate both your wrists externally
so that the hands are pointing outwards.

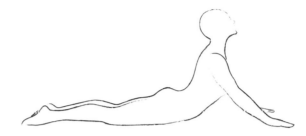

4 Engage the abdominal muscles even more strongly as you push into the hands to float the forearms off the floor.

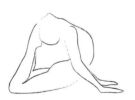

5 If there is any pain or a nervy sensation in the lower back, come straight back into sphinx pose. Otherwise, stay and breathe in seal pose, dropping the shoulders away from the ears. To intensify the pose further you could experiment with bending one or both knees, and even drop your head backward to meet your toes, if you're able.

6 When you are ready to come out, lower all the way back to the ground, bringing the big toes to touch and heels to fall apart. Make a pillow with your hands and turn your face to one direction to rest against them.

Camel

ustrasana

The full version of camel pose is a strong back bend that should only be attempted if you are properly warmed up and injury free. Both baby and half camel are good alternatives if you are still working on your back flexibility.

Camel pose does not have ancient origins – at least not documented ones – being first recorded in twentieth-century texts, including by K. Pattabhi Jois and B.K.S. Iyengar. The explanations given for the name are varied, including the arched front body in this posture resembling a camel's hump; the kneeling position being similar to how camels fold their legs to sit; and even the ponderous, steady (if surprisingly fast!) motion of camels being similar to the patience needed to build up to doing this pose. Camels are incredibly well evolved to survive in their native environment. While camel pose might initially feel very unnatural, having an awareness of your own ability to survive and thrive may bring another dimension to the practice of the posture.

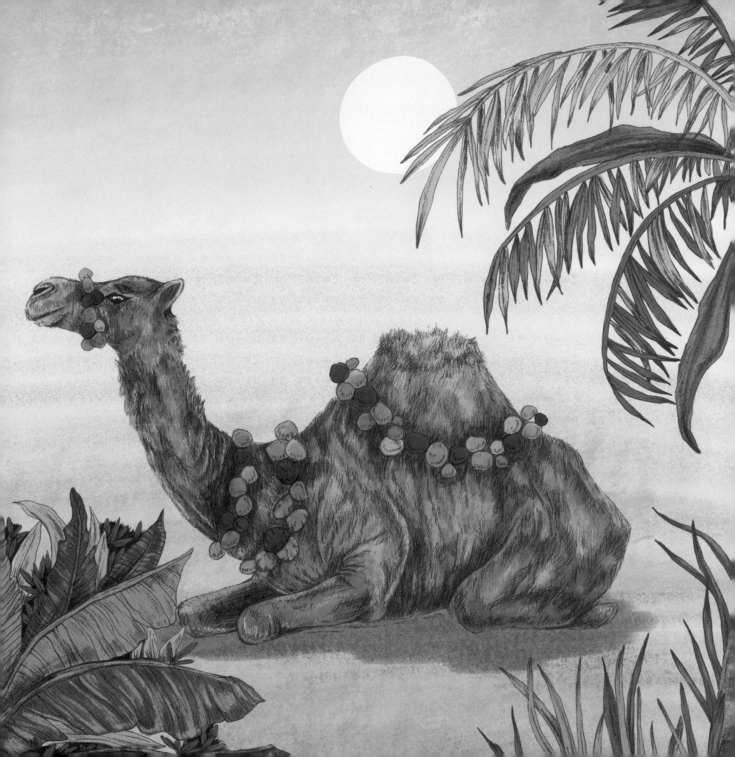

Camel Pose Step by step

As well as both stretching and strengthening the back, camel pose stretches into the shoulders, chest, throat and the quadriceps muscles.

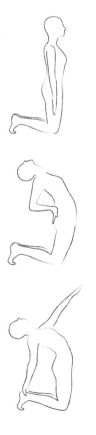

1 Come to kneel upright with hip points directly above knees. Tuck the toes under – you may need to manually tuck the baby toes. You can cushion the knees by doubling up the mat or putting a folded blanket underneath them.

2 Bring the hands to the mid back, fingers pointing down the back, elbows drawing towards each other. This is baby camel, or camel prep, and you can work here for as long as is necessary, opening into the chest and softening the hip flexors at the front.

3 If you're ready to go further, you can move to half camel (*ardha ustrasana*), taking your right hand to your right heel, with the left arm reaching forward at shoulder height, and then swapping arms. Keep moving in this way, synchronizing the movement with the breath in a little flow.

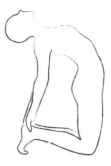

4 To come to full camel pose, reach both hands back to the respective heels. Keep the hips stacked above the knees, softening the hip flexors. Stay here and breathe.

5 To come out, reach one arm forward, then the second. Rest in child's pose (for a reminder, see p 80).

6 Repeat, or – to come further – untuck the toes and then bring the hands back to the heels for a stronger expression of the pose.

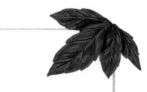

Not quite ready for camel pose?

Work on your back bending in bow pose (*dhanurasana*).

Dolphin

ardha pincha mayurasana or *catur svanasana*

Dolphin pose is a brilliant way of building strength in the arms, shoulders and core muscles while also stretching the hamstrings and shoulders, and, at the same time, getting all the benefits of an inversion. It is often used as a preparatory pose for postures such as headstand (*sirsasana*) or feathered peacock (*pincha mayurasana*).

The English name 'dolphin' is usually understood to refer to the clasped-hand position resembling that sea creature's bottlenose. However, as you flow powerfully back and forth you might think of a dolphin leaping playfully through the waves, and you can bring a sense of fun to the practice of this pose.

Inversions

Inversions encourage the flow of deoxygenated blood towards the heart and lungs, as well as oxygenated blood to the brain and sensory organs of the head. They also take weight off the feet and legs. Depending on the pose they can be energizing or restorative, and can bring a huge sense of achievement. Even humble poses such as downward-facing dog count as an inversion, as it raises the heart above the head.

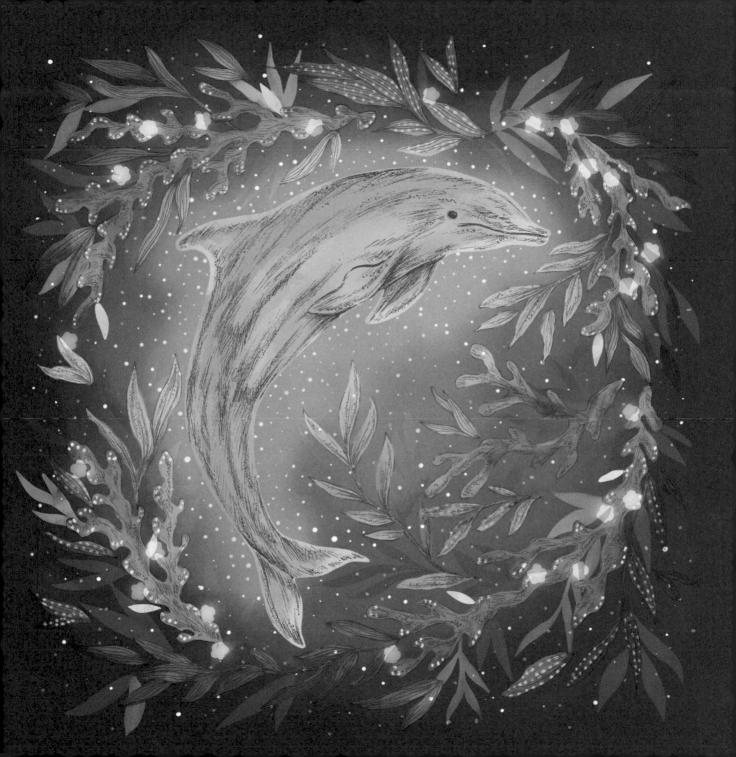

Dolphin Pose Step by step

It can be practised either as a static forearm downward-facing dog variation, or as a flow between this and a forearm plank variation, the latter being especially good for building heat and strength in the body.

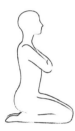

1 Come to kneel on the middle of your mat with the web of your hands snuggled into the crook of the opposite elbow.

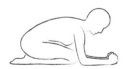

2 Maintaining this hand position, lower the elbows to the ground in front of your knees and then, keeping the same distance between them, open the forearms just enough to clasp the hands, palms together.

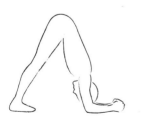

3 Tuck the toes under and lift the hips. This is a variation of downward dog. You can stay here and breathe, building strength and stamina.

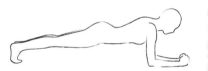

4 Otherwise, walk your feet back until you are in a forearm plank variation, body in a strong straight line. Drop the shoulders away from the ears and draw the abdominal muscles in. Engage the pelvic floor.

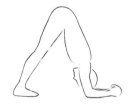

5 Inhale to lift the hips back into the forearm downward dog; exhale to lower back into the forearm plank. Repeat this nine more times or until you need a break.

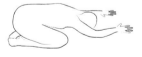

6 Rest in child's pose (for a reminder, see p 80).

7 Repeat this flow twice more.

Feathered Peacock & Scorpion
pincha mayurasana & vrischikasana

This pose is also often referred to in English as 'forearm stand' but 'feathered peacock' – the translation of the Sanskrit name – better conveys the heart-lifting beauty, flamboyance and grace of the posture. There can be a temptation to fling oneself up into or towards this pose without engaging the requisite muscles, running the risk of overbalancing. It might be beneficial to imagine a peacock calmly – casually, even – fanning its feathers, and trying to recreate that same considered, confident approach when coming into forearm stand.

Scorpion pose (*vrischikasana*) is an advanced back-bending variation of either handstand or forearm balance. Unless you are hypermobile in the back, this pose will take time and patience to build up to. The name comes from the shape the body makes – like a scorpion's tail curling over its body. Scorpions are known for being survivors in even the most hostile of circumstances. An ability to adapt is a crucial life skill and this spirit will serve you in scorpion pose.

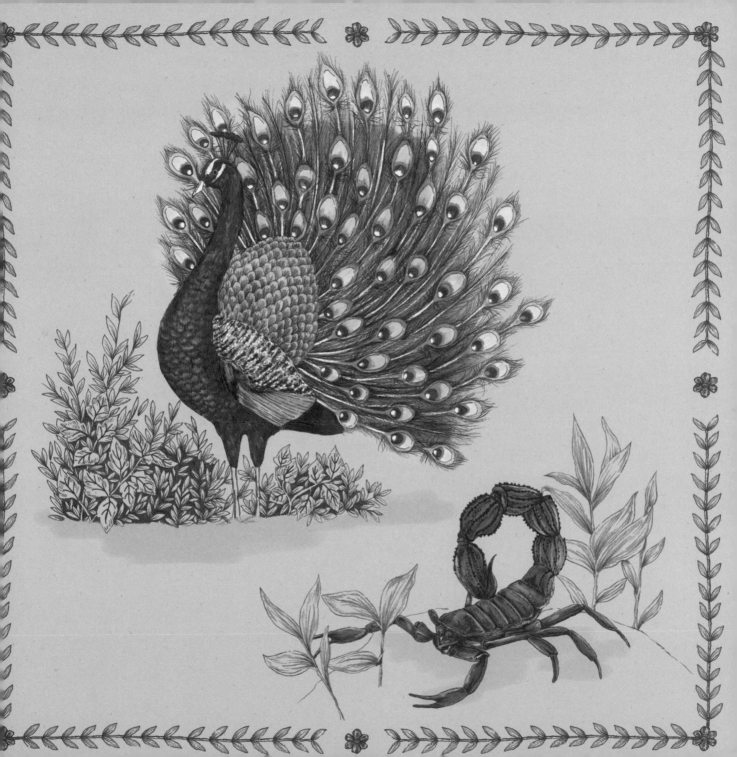

Feathered Peacock Pose Step by step

Like dolphin, which provides a route into peacock, this pose strengthens the muscles of the arms and shoulders, as well as the back, and also stretches into the shoulders and chest.

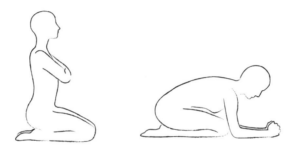

1 Begin in the same way as you did for dolphin, kneeling in the middle of the mat with the web of the hands hooked into the crook of the opposite elbows. Maintaining this position, bring the elbows to the floor in front of the knees.

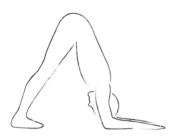

2 Now, keeping the elbows the same distance apart, open the forearms out to parallel. Plant the hands and spread the fingers.

3 Tuck the toes under and lift the hips towards the sky.

4 Tiptoe the feet closer towards the face until the hips are stacked over the shoulders. This should bring a tipping sensation of it almost being easier to lift the feet than keep them on the floor. A good rule of thumb is that this often involves the feet walking further towards the face than you initially think there is space for.

Feathered Peacock Pose Step by step

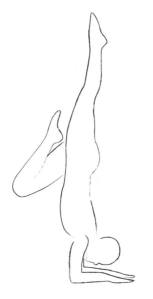

5 Experiment with extending one leg towards the sky. You can use the foot that is still on the ground to tip back and forth or even kick up gently. We tend to favour one leg for kicking up, so make sure you alternate which leg is lifted to build strength as evenly as possible. When the second leg lifts, bend the knee, moving the foot towards the buttock to help stabilize the pose.

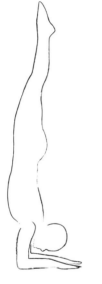

6 If you are able to lift both legs, carefully bring the inner thighs to hug together; keep the core muscles engaged and draw the front ribs in.

7 When you are ready to come out, lower down with control and then rest in child's pose (for a reminder, see p 80).

Scorpion Pose Step by step

This posture requires a strong opening into the chest and hollowing of the back, and shouldn't be attempted before you have mastered feathered peacock.

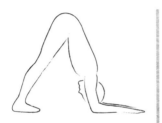

1 First, come into feathered peacock pose as described on p 112.

2 Keeping the frame of the shoulders strong and all four sides of the hands pressing firmly into the ground, begin to soften the chest forward between the arms.

3 When the chest has come forward as far as possible, start to bend the knees. You can let the legs separate somewhat, but bring the big toes to touch as they descend closer to your head.

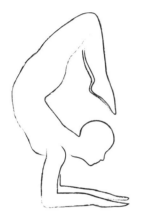

4 Keep the gaze forward and up and soften the back. Ease off or come out if there is any pinching sensation in the back.

5 To come down, first engage the core muscles and bring the legs together and back up into forearm balance. Bring the legs back to the ground with control.

6 Rest in child's pose (for a reminder, see p 80).

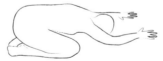

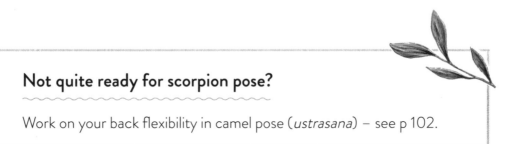

Not quite ready for scorpion pose?

Work on your back flexibility in camel pose (*ustrasana*) – see p 102.

Crow & Crane
kakasana & bakasana

Crow pose is one of the most accessible arm balances, and likely the first you will learn as a beginner. Crane looks very similar and can often be confused with crow pose – the key difference is that the arms are straight, whereas in crow pose the elbows are bent.

Crows are known to be adaptable and intelligent, while cranes are famous for their magnificent mating dances. These differences also apply to the poses, with crow being sturdier and crane more extravagant.

Arm balances

Many arm balances are also inversions and can form impressive shapes. They are strengthening poses, though often require more than just arm strength, and some depend upon flexibility, too. These poses can seem daunting. Above all, maintaining a sense of humour and perspective is key.

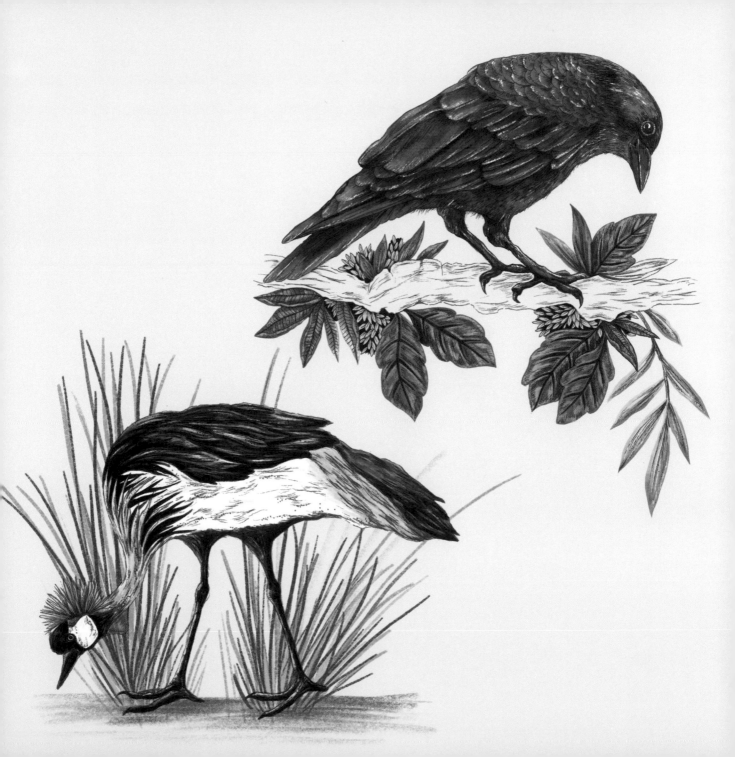

Crow & Crane Poses Step by step

The gaze (*drishti*) is important, as is remembering that you usually don't have far to fall. Those with strong arm muscles might find crow pose straightforward, but usually a mixture of arm and core strength, a steady gaze point, practice and a willingness to face and overcome the understandable fear of falling are all just as important.

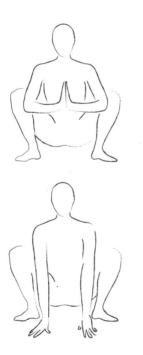

1 Come to a squat position with the feet about hip-distance apart, toes turning out.

2 Bring the hands to the floor shoulder-distance apart, fingers spread and pointing forward.

3 Come onto the balls of the feet and lift the bottom high.

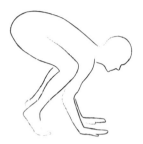

4 Bend the elbows, keeping the arms parallel,
and, at the same time, shift the weight forward
slowly, so that the knees come to the armpits or
upper triceps and the elbows stack above the
wrists. The arms are in the same position as they
are when lowering to the floor in yoga reverse
press-up (*chaturanga dandasana*), which makes
a handy shelf for the knees to brace against.

5 Look forward without crunching the neck –
if you look down, that's where you'll go!

Crow & Crane Pose Step by step

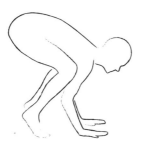

6 Play with tipping the weight forward so that just the big toes are touching the ground, then, engaging the muscles of the core, try lifting one big toe and then the other. You might stay here for your first several attempts, becoming attuned to your sense of balance.

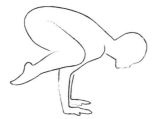

7 If you are able to lift both big toes from the ground, bring them to touch and then lift them towards the bottom. This is crow pose.

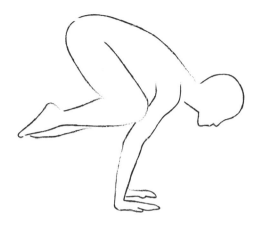

8 To turn your crow into a crane, work on getting the knees as far up the arms – and the arms as close to straight – as possible.

9 Stay in whichever variation you are in for a few breaths, then come out with control.

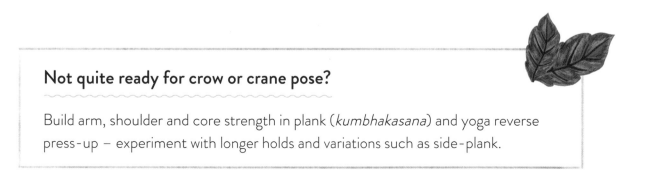

Not quite ready for crow or crane pose?

Build arm, shoulder and core strength in plank (*kumbhakasana*) and yoga reverse press-up – experiment with longer holds and variations such as side-plank.

Flying Pigeon
eka pada galavasana

The appearance of this pose may seem more like a perch
than flight (and the Sanskrit name may translate as 'one-legged
pose of [the sage] Galava', so nothing to do with birds),
but the feeling when you take off is no less than soaring.

It is not an accident that its English name is linked to the same
animal as one-legged king pigeon pose. In fact, the latter is
a very good exercise to prepare your hips for this big external
rotation. Despite their poor reputation in many quarters,
pigeons are among the most intelligent species of birds and
highly trainable. Approach your body in the same way,
coaching it into the pose with steadiness and persistence.

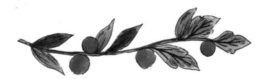

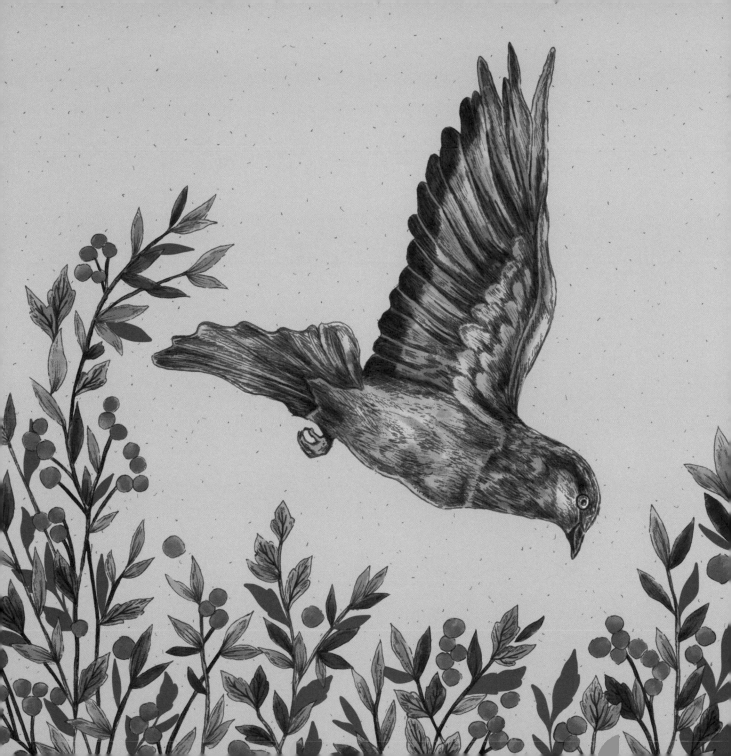

Flying Pigeon Pose Step by step

The position of the bent leg and the entry route described
below both require hip flexibility, and the pose works
to build strength in your arms, shoulders and core.

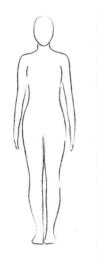

1 Come to stand in mountain pose
(*tadasana*), feeling rooted and grounded
in both feet and legs.

2 Before coming into the posture, first
warm up the hip and practise balancing
by taking the left foot into the right hand
and the left knee into the left hand. Rock
gently back and forth. As you begin to
soften into the hip you might be able to
take the left knee into the crook of the
left elbow, and the left foot into the crook
of the right elbow. Continue with the
gentle rocking motion.

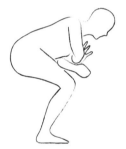

3 Now, cross the left ankle just above the right knee, flexing the left foot, and begin to bend the right leg until you are able to plant both hands firmly on the ground or blocks in front of you, shoulder distance apart.

4 Bend the elbows with the forearms parallel, as though you were lowering to the floor in yoga reverse press-up (*chaturanga dandasana*). Lean the left shin against the shelf of your upper arms and hook the left toes around the right triceps muscle, gripping firmly.

Flying Pigeon Pose Step by step

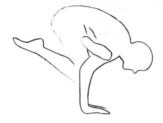

5 Look ahead of you on the floor and slowly shift your weight forward until your toes come off the floor. Tuck the right foot into the right buttock. If the pose is new to you, you may wish to stay here to explore and acclimatize. Push the floor away with your hands and broaden through the shoulder blades. Keep the core engaged.

6 When you are steady, experiment with extending the right leg, pushing through the ball of the foot while extending the chest in the opposite direction. There is also a version of the pose in which you extend energetically through the right leg, the ball of the foot pushing skywards. You could explore both, seeing if one is more accessible to you than the other.

7 Come out by carefully bringing both knees back
to the floor, then repeat with the other leg.

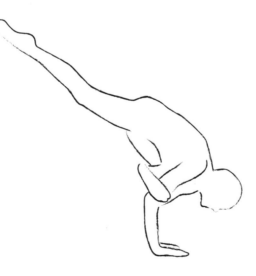

Elephant's Trunk & Firefly

eka hasta bhujasana & tittibhasana

This asymmetrical arm balance (the extended leg representing the elephant's trunk of the English name), requires flexibility in the hips as well as strength in the arms and core muscles. Elephants have the biggest brains of any land animals, and they are also capable of complex emotions and affection. The Sanskrit name of this pose literally means 'one hand shoulder/arm pose', but the English allows us to conjure the strength, stamina and perhaps also the sweet appeal of an elephant.

Firefly pose is a perfect example of an arm balance for which core strength is actually more important than that of the arm muscles. Its name comes from the Sanskrit word '*tittibha*' meaning 'firefly' or 'small insect'. Perhaps the outstretched legs represent the insect's wings or its antennae; maybe it's the hovering action of the pose that gives it its name; or perhaps it is the sense of magic associated with their famous bioluminescent glow that the pose will evoke for you.

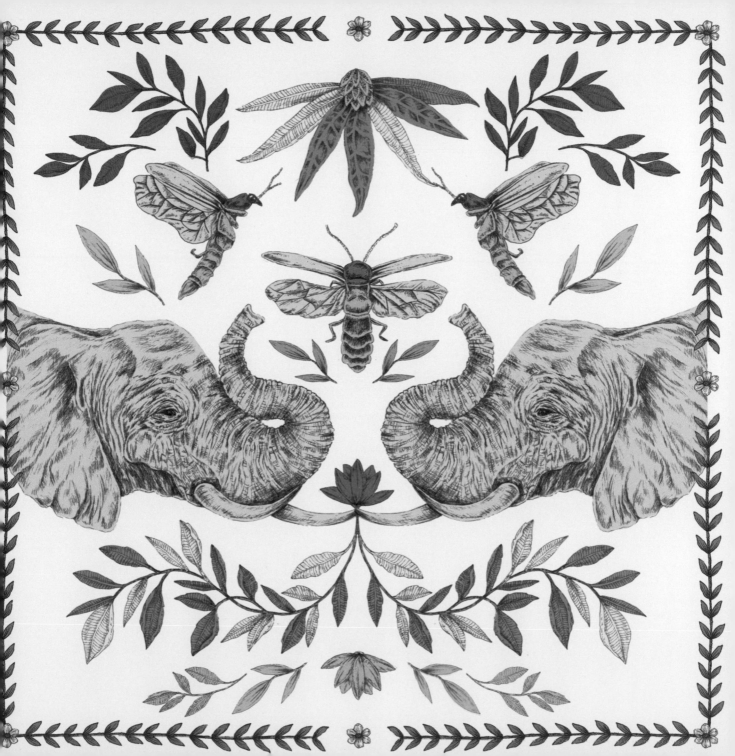

Elephant's Trunk Pose Step by step

This is a good pose to work on if firefly pose (see p 134–5) is not yet accessible to you, though it is still challenging in its own right.

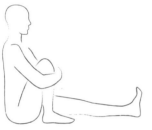

1 Come to sit on the ground with the legs together and outstretched, feet flexed.

2 Bend the right knee and hug it into the chest, foot planted on the floor.

3 Take the right arm inside the right leg, and behind the knee on the right thigh. Bring the right hand to the ground outside the right hip.

4 Bring the left hand to the floor outside the left hip and level with the right hand.

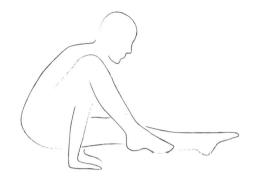

5 Engage the core, then push into the hands and the left heel to lift the bottom and the left leg off the floor. This may take time to work up to, but even the attempts help to tone and strengthen the relevant muscles.

6 Lower carefully to the floor and then repeat on the other side.

Firefly Pose Step by step

Firefly pose really requires all-round strength
and flexibility, so don't rush into it.

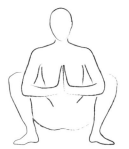

1 Bring the feet about shoulder-distance apart, or a little less, and come to a squat.

2 Work the torso between the legs as much as possible, then straighten the legs just enough so the pelvis comes to about hip height.

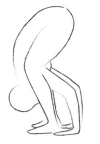

3 Take the left arm between the legs, wrapping it under the left thigh and around the outside of the left calf, putting the hand on the ground outside the left foot, fingers pointing forward. Repeat this action with the right arm and leg.

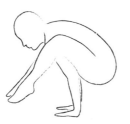

4 Engage your core muscles and lift up through the pelvic floor. Spread both hands and begin to press into them, squeezing your inner thighs against the upper arms and the arms back into the thighs at the same time.

5 Shift the weight from the feet onto the hands.

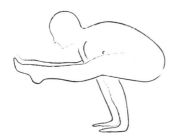

6 If you can, work to straighten the legs towards them being parallel with the ground, keeping the pelvis lifted.

7 To come out, slowly lower the legs and bottom back to the floor, then hug your knees into the body.

Peacock
mayurasana

When thinking of a peacock, we most often imagine one with tail feathers flamboyantly fanned as part of its mating ritual. It is often believed that peacocks are flightless birds but that is not the case, and it is a peacock's brief but triumphant aerial escapades that are channelled and honoured in this advanced arm-balancing pose. It is one of the oldest physical poses in hatha yoga to have been described and depicted – it is detailed, for example, in the *Hatha Yoga Pradipika*, and shown in a mural dating from around 1820. The peacock is sacred in Hindu mythology and is the national bird of India; it is a symbol of immortality and love, and peacock feathers are believed to have protective qualities.

Peacock pose is a great strengthener for the arms, wrists, core, legs and back muscles. It stimulates the abdominal organs and invigorates the whole body. When in the full pose, a yogi should resemble a peacock in flight, neck extended forward, legs representing the tail feathers furled and stretching in the opposite direction, arms tucked under like the bird's legs.

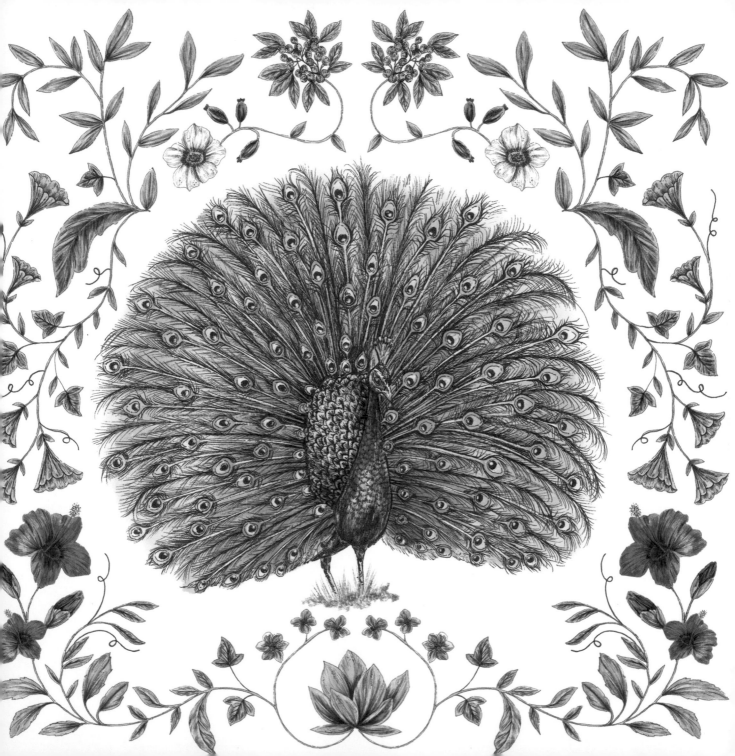

Peacock Pose Step by step

As with all dynamic or strong yoga poses, you should warm up thoroughly before attempting peacock pose. Sun salutations are good for a full-body stretch and warm-up. Do not attempt this pose if you have any wrist or elbow injuries.

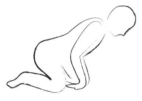

1 Come to a kneeling position with the knees wide, hands on the floor in front of you, fingers spread and pointing towards the body, outside edge of the little fingers touching.

2 Bend the elbows slightly so that their outer edges and those of the forearms touch, then keep bending until they are at a right angle.

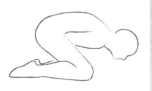

3 Slide the knees forward to outside and in front of the hands, and then tip the weight forward so that the abdomen rests against the triceps and the elbows dig into (or just below) the belly button.

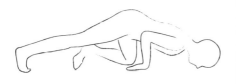

4 Bring the forehead to the floor and step the legs back one at a time until they are straight, with the tops of the feet pressing into the floor.

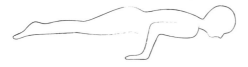

5 Engage the muscles of the abdomen against the elbows, and activate those of the legs and buttocks too. Lift the chest and head and look forward. Shift the weight slightly forward again to lift the legs and lengthen the whole body away from the floor. Stay here and breathe for five seconds, or as long as you can manage.

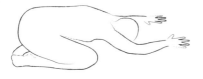

6 To come out, slowly lower the knees to the floor, take the weight off the hands and push back into child's pose (for a reminder, see p 80).

Not quite ready for peacock pose?

Build arm and core strength with plank pose and yoga reverse press-up. Build strength in your back muscles with locust pose (*salabhasana*).

Rooster
urdhva kukkutasana

This highly challenging arm balance requires open hips to come into lotus pose (*padmasana*) before you even consider the arm, shoulder, abdominal and chest strength to lift that lotus off the ground. It is also strengthening for the abdominal muscles and the hip flexors, and shouldn't be attempted before you are very comfortable in both lotus and crow poses. It involves lifting the head further from the ground than many other arm balances, so the risks attached to falling are somewhat greater.

The Sanskrit name translates as 'upward rooster', differentiating it from another variation of the pose. You might think of it as 'flying rooster', as the only part of the body that remains on the floor is the hands, the rest becoming airborne. Roosters are famed for their triumphant morning crowing – a verb used of humans to suggest boasting and strutting – and their flashy combs with which they attract mates. So, too, this pose, when achievable, is a chance to celebrate and show off what your amazing body can do!

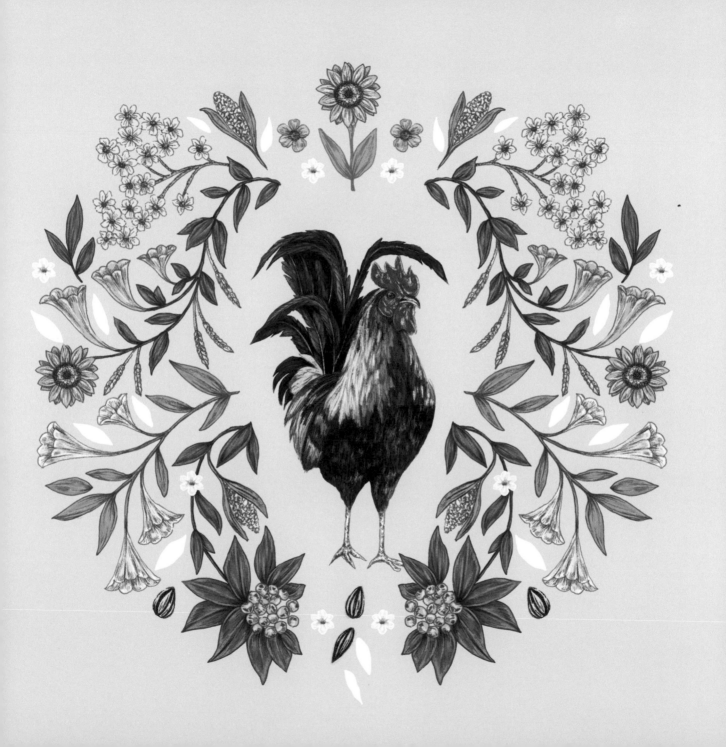

Rooster Pose Step by step

You may like to have a cushion in front of you in case of falling, but this is another reason to only attempt the pose when you feel properly prepared and have been practising yoga for some time.

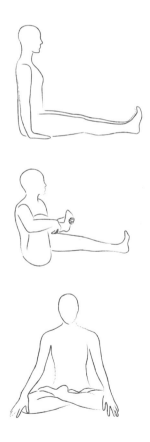

1 First prepare for lotus pose by warming up the hips. Come to sit with the legs outstretched.

2 Bend the right knee and hold it with the right hand, holding the right foot with the left hand and opening the knee out to the side. Rock the knee gently back and forth, priming the hip joint. As you begin to soften into the hip, you can snuggle the right knee into the right inner elbow, the foot into the left inner elbow, then continue this rocking motion. Repeat with the left leg.

3 Take the right foot in both hands and fold it into the left hip crease. Repeat with the left leg and the right hip crease.

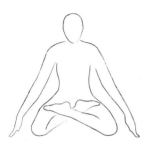

4 Now, maintaining the legs in lotus position, rock forward onto the knees and bring the hands to the floor so that your wrists are right in front of your knees, fingertips pointing forward.

5 Exhale, rounding the back and hollowing out the tummy.

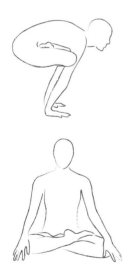

6 Inhale, and, engaging the core and lifting through the pelvic floor, begin to slide the knees up the back of the legs. This may take many breaths and many attempts! The aim is to get the knees up to the armpits, but you may not achieve this the first several times. Take it slowly and patiently.

7 Come out carefully and repeat with the other leg on top in lotus.

Fish

matsyasana

As with many back bends, fish pose can be energizing and mood-boosting. '*Matsya*' is the Sanskrit word for 'fish' and also an incarnation of the Hindu god Vishnu. Up to 60 per cent of the adult human body is composed of water. As you practise this pose, breathing into the big opening in the chest, you might like to imagine yourself floating among the waves, calm and at-home, come what may.

Winding down

The winding down portion of your yoga sessions is just as important as any other part and not to be skipped. On a purely physical level, we need to counter-stretch and cool down, iron out and check in on any sensations that might have arisen during our practice. But in terms of supporting our whole body-mind system, standing down the fight-or-flight response, lowering the heart rate and blood pressure, and boosting the secondary functions such as digestion is vital.

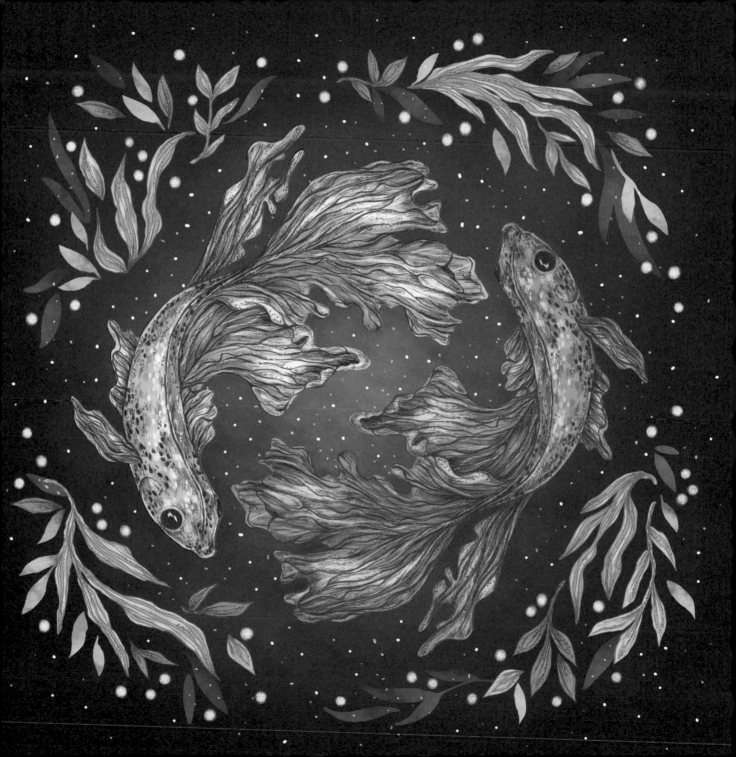

Fish Pose Step by step

Fish pose is often practised after inversions, especially shoulder stand (*salamba sarvangasana*) and plough pose (*halasana*), stretching and opening into the thoracic spine, neck, chest and shoulders.

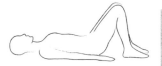

1 Come to lie on your back with the knees bent and above the ankles.

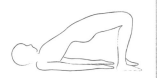

2 Inhale to lift the hips and bring the arms underneath the body, shoulders snuggled beneath you as far as possible. Hook the thumbs and pull the arms as straight as you can.

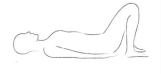

3 Lower the upper body onto the straight arms and release the hook of the thumbs.

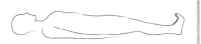

4 Walk the feet away from the view of the face until the legs are straight and together, feet flexed.

5 Inhale, pushing the elbows into the floor and puffing out the chest; lift the head and then lower the crown of it gently back onto the ground, so you are baring your throat to the ceiling. Let the mouth lightly close and keep pushing into the ground with the arms and legs to prevent there being too much pressure on the head. Don't turn the head while in this position.

6 Hold for several breaths, then lead with the puffing of the chest again to carefully lift then lower the back of the head to the floor.

7 Clasp the hands behind the head and use the strength of the arms to lift the head with care to look at the feet for a breath or two. Lower slowly to the ground.

Rabbit

sasangasana

Rabbit pose (also sometimes called 'hare pose') can be seen as a kind
of extension of child's pose, and is also technically an inversion, with
all the benefits that entails. Rabbits are famous for being fast, agile
and sociable. The name of this pose is usually said to come from the
position of the spine when practising it resembling that of a rabbit,
but you might also find the arm position reminiscent of its ears,
or even cultivate a little springiness in the body and mood as you
work to keep there from being too much weight on the head.
While this pose should be accessible for most, that isn't to say
it is *easy* necessarily. Use your breath to explore the posture
and be ready to ease off or come out if need be.

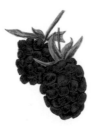

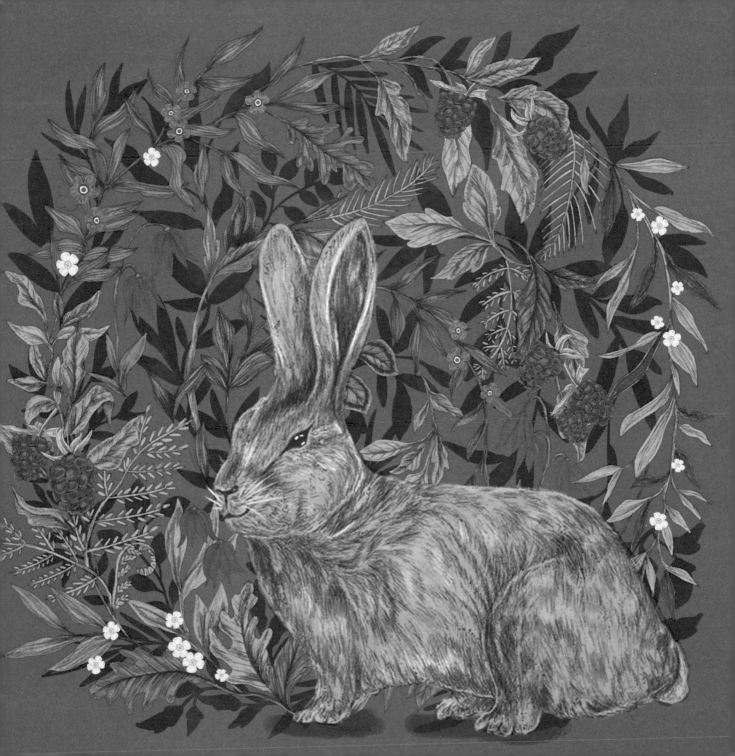

Rabbit Pose Step by step

Rabbit pose is a good stretch for the spine, shoulders and neck.

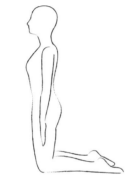

1 Come to kneel on the ground with the hip points stacked above the knees.

2 Take the hands to the floor shoulder-width apart, closer to the knees than they would be in all-fours position.

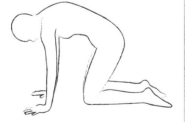

3 Inhale, letting the belly soften and round, then, as you exhale, draw the abdominal muscles in and up, hollowing the front body as you bring the crown of the head to the ground.

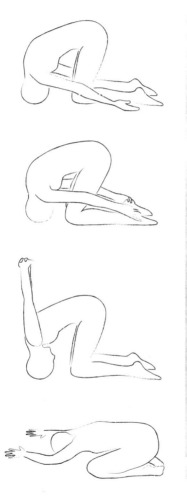

4 Walk the hands back and alongside the shins to take hold of the heels if possible.

5 Grip the heels firmly and push into the floor with the tops of the feet and shins to help keep the pressure on the top of the head light.

6 Stay here and breathe or, for a more intense shoulder stretch, clasp the hands together on the tailbone and then breathe them up and over in an arc towards the head. This makes them look especially like a rabbit's ears!

7 To come out, sit back on the heels in child's pose (for a reminder, see p 80).

Crocodile
makarasana

This pose really embodies the spirit of full rest as described in 'winding down' on p 144. It could be used as an alternative to corpse pose (*savasana* – see p 156–9) that opens into the shoulders and upper back, and helps to release tension in the lower back. The Sanskrit word '*makara*' has been translated as 'crocodile', 'dolphin' and even 'sea monster'; however, in this flat position it is easy to picture a crocodile lurking, only eyes, ears and nostrils visible above the surface of the water, perfectly still and conserving its energy for when it is most needed. Crocodiles can be associated with wisdom and renewal – ideal symbols for this pose of conscious and deliberate rest.

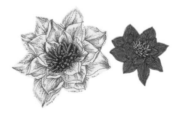

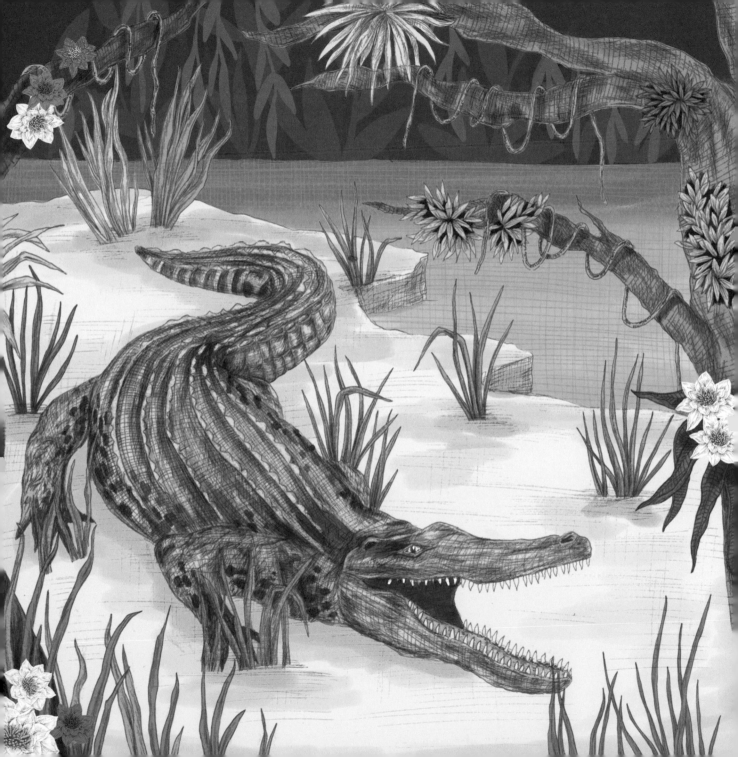

Crocodile Pose Step by step

This pose allows you to breathe deeply
into the back of the lungs.

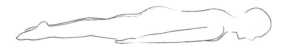

1 Come to lie face down on the ground, legs extended
and wider than hip-distance apart.

2 Make a pillow with the hands and bring the forehead
to rest on them.

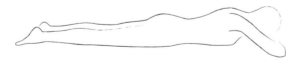

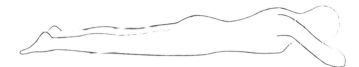

3 Scan the whole body from feet to head, noticing anywhere that you might be gripping or experiencing tension and sending your breath there to release it.

4 You could take your final relaxation in this position. Otherwise, stay here for several breaths at least, before pushing carefully back up to all fours.

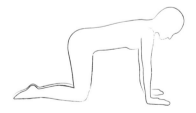

Corpse

savasana

This is the pose most commonly assumed for the final relaxation in a yoga session. It involves lying on the back, keeping completely still (or as close to that as possible). The instructor may lead the class in a guided meditation, or a yogi practising on their own might consciously relax each part of the body in turn.

The key is to relax deeply and fully without falling asleep – and this can be much trickier than it sounds. Beginner yogis might struggle to tune out the chattering of the mind, running through to-do lists or rehearsing conversations; or, on the other hand, they might instantly fall asleep! However, practising corpse pose at the end of a yoga session is the ideal time, as the body should be stretched and strengthened, the breathing deep and full. And with regular practice, the benefits of this deceptively complex pose will be ever more readily accessible. Despite the somewhat morbid-sounding name, when you find that sweet spot in corpse pose it can feel blissful and deeply restorative.

Corpse Pose Step by step

You can use blankets, bolsters, cushions or other props to make your final relaxation luxuriously comfortable, but, unless you require specific support or modifications, all you really need is the ground beneath you.

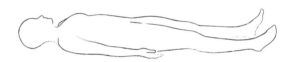

1 Come to lie flat on your back with your feet mat-width apart, toes turning out and arms alongside the body. If there is any discomfort in the lower back, you may prefer to bend the knees, take the feet mat-width apart and let the knees knock together.

2 Tense or squeeze and then relax each part of the body in turn: feet and legs; buttocks and hips; hands and arms; shoulder blades together; shoulders towards and then away from the ears; face, making it first into a prune, then opening mouth and eyes wide.

3 Make any adjustments or fidgets you need to in order to come to complete stillness.

4 Release any effort with the breath – let it soften; allow the eyes to gently close.

5 Take the mind on a tour of the body, relaxing each part in turn. You could silently even say to yourself, for example, 'I relax my right big toe, other four toes, ball of the foot, heel, top of the foot, ankle. My whole right foot is completely relaxed,' repeating this with each part of the body all the way to the top of the head. If the mind wanders, try not to attach any feelings to that – simply call it back to the body and the breath.

6 Relax the whole mind and body.

7 Stay here for as long as you can but try to allow at least two full minutes (ten would be better).

8 Come out very gradually. First, take your awareness to the sounds of your own body: breath, heartbeat, pulse. Next, take your awareness to the sounds of the room around you; then the building around that. Finally, take your awareness all the way to the outside world – the furthest-away sounds you can detect.

9 Keeping the eyes closed, reintroduce movement to the body slowly, beginning by gently wriggling fingers and toes, then rolling the head gently from side to side.

10 When you're ready, stretch in whatever way feels good to you now.

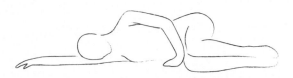

11 Still with your eyes closed, roll carefully on to one side with the top hand on the floor, reconnecting to that grounding energy. Use that top hand to push yourself up to a seated position.

12 Rub the hands together to create some warmth, then take the hands over the closed eyes. Separate the fingers to let a little light in, blink the eyes open and finally remove the hands from the eyes.

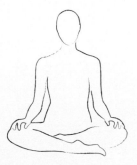

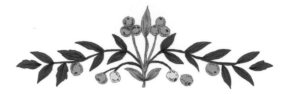

Emily Sharratt is an editor, writer and qualified yoga instructor. She has been teaching for over eight years, as well as having a regular practice for almost twenty. Her teaching method encompasses a range of yoga styles, from vinyasa flow to yin, and she considers the final relaxation the most important part of a class.

Emily's favourite yoga animal pose is *eka pada rajakapotasana* (one-legged king pigeon), but she also enjoys working on her *eka pada galavasana* (flying pigeon) and *pincha mayurasana* (feathered peacock). Emily lives in London with her daughter, whose favourite yoga pose is a three-legged downward-facing dog-headstand hybrid of her own invention.

Jade Mosinski is a Derbyshire-based designer and illustrator who loves to create beautiful and intricate illustrations inspired by the natural world, using detailed line work. She has designed cards and wrap sold in John Lewis, Paperchase and Waterstones, and the Jade Mosinski Designs range of greeting cards for Blue Eyed Sun is an expanding collection of over 100 designs.

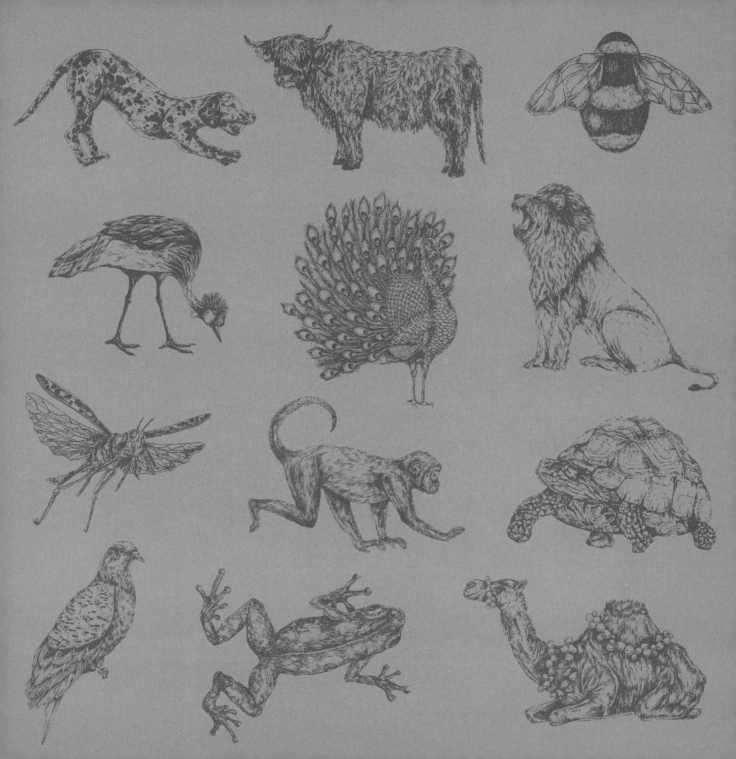